LOW POWER ANALOG CMOS FOR CARDIAC PACEMAKERS

THE KLUWER INTERNATIONAL SERIES IN ENGINEERING AND COMPUTER SCIENCE

ANALOG CIRCUITS AND SIGNAL PROCESSING
Consulting Editor: Mohammed Ismail. *Ohio State University*

Related Titles:

MIXED-SIGNAL LAYOUT GENERATION CONCEPTS
Lin, van Roermund, Leenaerts
ISBN: 1-4020-7598-7
HIGH-FREQUENCY OSCILLATOR DESIGN FOR INTEGRATED TRANSCEIVERS
Van der Tang, Kasperkovitz and van Roermund
ISBN: 1-4020-7564-2
CMOS INTEGRATION OF ANALOG CIRCUITS FOR HIGH DATA RATE TRANSMITTERS
DeRanter and Steyaert
ISBN: 1-4020-7545-6
SYSTEMATIC DESIGN OF ANALOG IP BLOCKS
Vandenbussche and Gielen
ISBN: 1-4020-7471-9
SYSTEMATIC DESIGN OF ANALOG IP BLOCKS
Cheung & Luong
ISBN: 1-4020-7466-2
LOW-VOLTAGE CMOS LOG COMPANDING ANALOG DESIGN
Serra-Graells, Rueda & Huertas
ISBN: 1-4020-7445-X
CIRCUIT DESIGN FOR WIRELESS COMMUNICATIONS
Pun, Franca & Leme
ISBN: 1-4020-7415-8
DESIGN OF LOW-PHASE CMOS FRACTIONAL-N SYNTHESIZERS
DeMuer & Steyaert
ISBN: 1-4020-7387-9
MODULAR LOW-POWER, HIGH SPEED CMOS ANALOG-TO-DIGITAL CONVERTER FOR EMBEDDED SYSTEMS
Lin, Kemna & Hosticka
ISBN: 1-4020-7380-1
DESIGN CRITERIA FOR LOW DISTORTION IN FEEDBACK OPAMP CIRCUITE
Hernes & Saether
ISBN: 1-4020-7356-9
CIRCUIT TECHNIQUES FOR LOW-VOLTAGE AND HIGH-SPEED A/D CONVERTERS
Walteri
ISBN: 1-4020-7244-9
DESIGN OF HIGH-PERFORMANCE CMOS VOLTAGE CONTROLLED OSCILLATORS
Dai and Harjani
ISBN: 1-4020-7238-4
CMOS CIRCUIT DESIGN FOR RF SENSORS
Gudnason and Bruun
ISBN: 1-4020-7127-2
ARCHITECTURES FOR RF FREQUENCY SYNTHESIZERS
Vaucher
ISBN: 1-4020-7120-5
THE PIEZOJUNCTION EFFECT IN SILICON INTEGRATED CIRCUITS AND SENSORS
Fruett and Meijer
ISBN: 1-4020-7053-5
CMOS CURRENT AMPLIFIERS; SPEED VERSUS NONLINEARITY
Koli and Halonen
ISBN: 1-4020-7045-4
MULTI-STANDARD CMOS WIRELESS RECEIVERS
Li and Ismail
ISBN: 1-4020-7032-2

LOW POWER ANALOG CMOS FOR CARDIAC PACEMAKERS

Design and Optimization in Bulk and SOI Technologies

by

Fernando Silveira

Universidad de la República and CCC S.A.,
Montevideo, Uruguay

and

Denis Flandre

Université catholique de Louvain,
Louvain-la-Neuve, Belgium

KLUWER ACADEMIC PUBLISHERS

BOSTON / DORDRECHT / LONDON

A C.I.P. Catalogue record for this book is available from the Library of Congress.

ISBN 978-1-4419-5419-0

Published by Kluwer Academic Publishers,
P.O. Box 17, 3300 AA Dordrecht, The Netherlands.

Sold and distributed in North, Central and South America
by Kluwer Academic Publishers,
101 Philip Drive, Norwell, MA 02061, U.S.A.

In all other countries, sold and distributed
by Kluwer Academic Publishers,
P.O. Box 322, 3300 AH Dordrecht, The Netherlands.

Printed on acid-free paper

Contents

Contents

Acknowledgements

This book and the work that is presented in it would not have been possible without the technical, practical, financial and encouraging support that was provided by many individuals and institutions.

We are deeply grateful to Prof. Paul Jespers, who is at the origin of the relationship of Fernando Silveira with the Université catholique de Louvain (UCL) and who sowed the seed for one of the mainstays of this work, the g_m/I_D method.

We want to thank the members of our labs: the Instituto de Ingeniería Eléctrica at Universidad de la República (UR) and the Microelectronics Laboratory at UCL, for making them very enjoyable places of work.

At UCL, we must particularly point out the helping hand of the following people: Anne Adant, Xavier Baie, Jian Chen, André Crahay, Laurent Demeûs, Vincent Dessard, Carlos Dualibe, Brigitte Dupont, Jean-Paul Eggermont, Luiz Ferreira, Bernard Gentinne, Benjamín Iñiguez, Bernard Herent, Pierre Loumaye and Alberto Viviani.

At UR we want to thank all the members of the Microelectronics Group, who worked with F. Silveira on the design and test of the industrial pacemaker chip: Alfredo Arnaud, Marcelo Barú, Oscar de Oliveira, Pablo Mazzara, Gonzalo Picún, Conrado Rossi and the late Hugo Valdenegro. We specially acknowledge the key participation of some members of the group in other works that are part of this book: the contribution of Alfredo Arnaud in the development of the model of the sample and hold presented in Appendix 2; the participation of Oscar de Oliveira and Conrado Rossi in, respectively, the initial development of the switched capacitor sense channel and its layout, and the participation of Linder Reyes in the test of this circuit. We also thank the students Leonardo Díaz and Ricardo Clavijo for their work on the layout and simulation of the amplifier A4 presented in Chapter 5. F. Silveira is indebted to Facultad de Ingeniería and the Instituto de Ingeniería Eléctrica (IIE) for supporting the development of his thesis, particularly the head of his department, Prof. Rafael Canetti and the head of the IIE, Prof. Gregory Randall.

The development of the central subject of this book was possible due to the collaboration with CCC del Uruguay S.A. F. Silveira is thankful to those that took the decision of working with UR in this area; Julio Arzuaga, Fernando Brum, Alicia Fiandra and Orestes Fiandra. He is also very grateful to Julio Arzuaga, Pedro Arzuaga and the rest of the members of CCC for their technical guidance in the field of pacemakers and medical implants, and for sharing their solid and wise approach to engineering problems.

We also wish to acknowledge the financial support of the Secrétariat à la Coopération Internationale at UCL, and the always warm and effective assistance of Mrs. Louise Baeyens, as well as financial support of the CSIC of UR and Conicyt of Uruguay in various projects related to this work.

We thank the members of the PhD thesis jury that contributed with valuable suggestions that helped to improve the thesis text that is the basis for this book: Profs. José Luis Huertas, Jean Didier Legat, Damien Macq and Michel Verleysen

We thank María del Carmen Aguado, for her help in checking and improving the language of this text and Laura Landing for her help in the formatting of the text.

Finally, and specially from our hearts, we are grateful to our families and friends, who endured our dedication to this work.

Preface

Power reduction is a central priority in battery-powered medical implantable devices, particularly pacemakers, to either increase battery lifetime or decrease size using a smaller battery. This book proposes new techniques for the reduction of power consumption in analog integrated circuits applied in pacemakers. Its main case of study is the pacemaker sense channel, which is representative of a broader class of biomedical circuits aimed at qualitatively detecting biological signals.

The book is expected to be useful for researchers, postgraduate students and designers in both the areas of analog integrated circuits and implantable medical devices.

The basis of this text was written as a Ph.D. thesis at the Université Catholique de Louvain, Louvain-la-Neuve, Belgium. Part of the work was developed at the Instituto de Ingeniería Eléctrica, Universidad de la República, Montevideo, Uruguay. Concurrently with the development of the thesis, an industrial integrated circuit for pacemakers was designed for CCC S.A, Uruguay, a pacemaker factory. In this and subsequent projects with CCC S.A. the pacemaker appeared as an example of choice for the analysis of the impact of application of SOI technology and power-aware design techniques.

The book contains six chapters. The first and second chapters are a tutorial presentation on implantable medical devices and pacemakers from the circuit designer point of view. This is illustrated by the requirements and solutions applied in our implementation of an industrial IC for pacemakers. Therefrom, the book discusses the means for reduction of power consumption at three levels: integration technology, power-oriented analytical synthesis procedures and circuit architecture.

At the technology level, we analyze the impact that the application of the fully depleted silicon-on-insulator (FD SOI) CMOS technology has on this kind of analog circuits. The basic building block level as well as the system level (pacemaker sense channel) are considered.

Concerning the design technique, we apply a methodology, based on the transconductance to current ratio, that exploits all regions of inversion of the MOS transistor. Various performance aspects of analog building blocks are modeled and a power optimization synthesis of OTAs for a given total settling time (including the slewing and linear regions) is proposed.

At the circuit level, we present a new design approach of a class AB output stage suitable for micropower application. In our design approach, the usual advantages of the application of a class AB output stage are enhanced by the application of a transconductance multiplication effect.

These techniques are tested in experimental prototypes of amplifiers and complete pacemaker sense channel implementations in SOI and standard bulk CMOS technologies.

A ultra low consumption of 110 nA (0.3 μW) is achieved in a FD SOI sense channel implementation.

Though primarily addressed to the pacemaker system, the techniques proposed are shown to have application in other contexts where power reduction is a main concern.

Next, we present an outline of the content of each chapter.

Chapter 1 Implantable Cardiac Pacemakers.

The first chapter provides the reader with the main framework set by the target application and the general specifications that this application imposes on the circuits studied in this work.

The chapter is organized in three parts. In the first part, we introduce a brief view of the operation and functionality of modern implantable cardiac pacemakers at the system level. The second part describes the circuit blocks that are comprised in these devices and the requirements imposed on some of these circuit blocks, while reviewing the prior published work on implantable pacemaker circuit design. Finally, in the third part, we show, by the analysis of other medical devices and functions, that the essential requirements of the pacemaker sense amplifier are common to several devices, allowing the conclusions of our study to have wider application.

Chapter 2 Industrial Implementation of Pacemaker Integrated Circuit in Bulk CMOS Technology.

The second chapter discusses the architectural alternatives, trade-offs, actual design and results of circuits we have implemented in Bulk CMOS technology, for a pacemaker's analog processing functions. Particularly we focused on two main analog modules of a pacemaker: the sense channel and the activity sense block.

The analysis of this industrial design provides us with detailed specifications and performance data that will be later applied to design and to evaluate alternative architectures and technology (SOI). In addition, the methods applied to meet the challenges of operation of analog circuits at low-voltage (2V) power supply in a standard Bulk CMOS process are described.

Regarding the design of the sense channel, the selection of the overall architecture and the main design characteristics of the basic building blocks are presented. In particular the compromise between the use of external components and the implementation of a fully integrated solution is discussed. A review of the alternatives for integrated implementation of large time constants is presented in the Appendix 1 of the book.

As an additional example of micropower analog block of the pacemaker, the design of an accelerometer signal conditioning circuit for activity sensing is presented in the Appendix 2 of the book.

Chapter 3. Potential of SOI Technology for Low-Voltage Micropower Biomedical Applications.

The goal of the third chapter is to introduce the reader to the characteristics of Fully-Depleted (FD) SOI technology and to evaluate its potential impact in biomedical applications that require analog blocks under low-voltage operation and micropower consumption.

The chapter starts by briefly reviewing the features of the FD SOI technology. Then, we analyze the improvements that can be obtained for the operation of basic components such as analog switches, current mirrors and operational transconductance amplifiers (OTAs). These analyses devote particular attention to those blocks and performance aspects that are central to the proposed implementation of our study vehicle, the sense channel, as well as to the implementation of other pacemaker analog blocks. This is the case of the speed and precision of current mirrors, which are essential elements in the class AB stage proposed in Chapter 5, and of OTA characteristics such as the power – bandwidth trade-off, noise and offset.

Chapter 4. Power optimization in operational amplifier design.

The fourth chapter is aiming at shedding light on the ultimate reasons that condition power consumption in amplifier design. An analysis of the factors that determine power consumption leads us on to the selection of the most effective ways to reduce it. The results are then applied to the power optimization of a Miller operational transconductance amplifier (OTA).

In the first part, we present a brief review of existing results about theoretical limits of power consumption of analog circuits. These results suggest the essential mechanisms to get closer to these limits; they serve as comparison reference and they identify the criteria on the formulation of figures of merit for comparison between actual circuit implementations. The first part ends with a review of the practical limits and the introduction of a general scheme of the factors that determine power consumption in operational amplifiers. The results presented in this first part, besides its interest from the general point of view of low-power analog design, provide elements required in order to perform a fair comparison of the results of our amplifiers and the pacemaker sense channel with other published amplifiers and filters.

The second part formulates a "power oriented" synthesis of the Miller OTA. We introduce a new procedure to handle the trade-off between linear settling time (associated to the gain-bandwidth product) and slew rate, which applies a novel, joint optimization of these two aspects to achieve minimum power consumption. The proposed design procedure, which can be extended to other OTA architectures, makes it possible to determine numerically the best combination of the input and output stage g_m/I_D ratio and simultaneously provides insight on the underlying reasons that lead to this optimum.

Chapter 5. Class AB Micropower Operational Amplifiers.

The fifth chapter presents a novel design approach for a class AB output stage, as required to save quiescent power in the pacemaker sense channel.

The chapter is organized as follows. First, we introduce the general characteristics of class AB stages and review the main structures found in the literature. Then, we describe the selected architecture and the method applied to synthesize it for minimum power consumption. Next, the experimental results on the fabricated prototypes and comparisons with reported amplifiers of similar characteristic are presented. Finally, improvements to the basic circuit structure and design method are discussed.

Chapter 6. Implementation of pacemaker sense circuits.

The last chapter describes the application of various techniques and ideas developed in the book to the design of pacemaker sense circuits. First we present a switched capacitor (SC) design of a sense channel filter / amplifier in 0.8μm Bulk technology. Next, we describe a continuous time implementation of the sense channel in FD SOI technology that achieves a ultra low consumption of only 110nA, applying the general architecture described in Chapter 2.

Finally, the main conclusions and future research lines are summarized.

Chapter 1

Implantable Cardiac Pacemakers

Microelectronic technology is steadily contributing to the development of medical therapies and diagnostic aids. Many of these developments follow the general trend towards low-power and low-voltage circuits of electronic systems, in order to satisfy the voltage requirements of sub-micron technologies, as well as the need for portable terminals and heat dissipation management in complex chips. Nevertheless, the medical device field where the quest for realizing minimum consumption circuits and devices has been the most intense is still the area of active implantable devices.

Implantable devices are defined as those intended to be surgically placed inside the body and remain there for a long term. The active quality refers to devices that have a power supply and are capable of delivering energy to the body, in contrast with passive implants like metallic bone prostheses.

Most of the active implantable devices in current application are powered by batteries. Since their replacement requires a surgical procedure, though simple in most cases, the need arises for minimizing power consumption to increase device lifetime. Few exceptions exist where the system is powered by RF energy transmitted from the outside of the body. Nevertheless, this is not always practical and consumption, though higher levels are allowed, is still an important concern.

The main example of active implantable device in terms of widespread application is the cardiac pacemaker.

In this book, one of the cardiac pacemaker circuit modules (the sense amplifier) will be used as a study vehicle for the application of low-power circuit techniques and SOI technology.

In the first section of this chapter, we introduce a brief system level survey of the operation and functionality of modern implantable cardiac pacemakers. The objective of this description is to provide the reader with

1

the main framework in which the circuits studied in this work will be included.

In section 2, we describe the circuit blocks of these devices and the requirements imposed on some of them, while reviewing prior published work on implantable pacemaker circuit design.

Finally in section 3, we show, by the analysis of other medical devices and functions, that key requirements of the pacemaker sense amplifier are common to several devices, allowing the conclusions of our study to have wider application.

1.   THE HEART AND IMPLANTABLE CARDIAC PACEMAKERS

A cardiac pacemaker reestablishes a normal rhythm to a diseased heart that basically presents a slower contraction rate or similar disorders. In order to give an overall view of the pacemaker operation, we firstly present a very brief summary of the heart operation based on [WEB951].

1.1   The Heart Operation

The human heart consists of two pumps in series, one to propel blood through the lungs for exchange of oxygen and carbon dioxide and the other to propel blood to all other tissues of the body. Figure 1-1 depicts the blood flow in a schematic way.

The ventricles are the main pumps and the atria are auxiliary pumps that function as filling and holding chambers while the ventricles contract. A valve system assures the unidirectional flow of the blood.

The structure and behavior of the heart muscles, as well as the way the contraction of the heart chambers is commanded, determine many important characteristics of the operation of both heart and pacemaker. The cardiac musculature consists of two types of muscle cells: (1) cells that initiate and conduct impulses, and (2) cells that besides conducting, respond to stimuli by contracting. The latter constitute the working musculature of the heart or the myocardium. In the myocardium of the ventricles the cells are not electrically insulated or mechanically separated from one another. A stimulus arising at any point in the ventricle spreads to cause complete contraction of both ventricular chambers. The same applies to the atria. The atria and ventricles are not connected except for the atrioventricular (AV) node, which is responsible for transmitting the contraction order from the atria to the ventricles. The sequence of excitation of the heart normally proceeds from the sinoatrial node, located on top of the atria, which is the natural pacemaker of the heart. The excitation spreads through both atria to the AV node, passing then on to the ventricles.

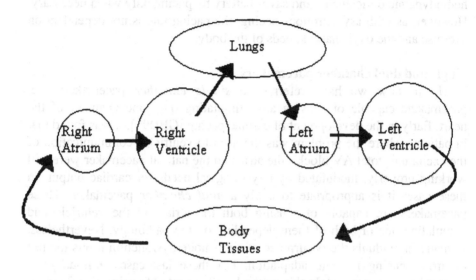

Figure 1-1. Schematic diagram of heart blood flow

1.2 Artificial Pacemaker Operation and Functionality

The main function of artificial pacemakers is to supply lacking excitation pulses from the sinoatrial node or to reestablish a malfunctioning excitation communication from the atria to the ventricles.

Asynchronous and synchronous pacing

Since the main pumping action is performed by the ventricles, the first generation of implantable cardiac pacemakers just stimulated the ventricles at a fixed rate [GED90] (*asynchronous pacing*). This type of operation has various drawbacks: the synchronicity between the atria and the ventricles may be lost thus decreasing the pumping efficiency, the rate is not dependent on exercise, and battery energy is being wasted in periods of correct functioning of the natural pacemaker system when external stimulation would not be necessary. Furthermore, in some patients this may cause fibrillation (a state of irregular contraction of the heart that can lead to death) if the pulse is delivered within the vulnerable period.

An early improvement of pacemakers was to incorporate the capacity of sensing events that correspond to the spontaneous contraction of the ventricles and inhibit the delivery of a stimulation pulse. This is called *synchronous or demand pacing*. If the searched-after event is not sensed within a time-out period, a pulse is delivered. This avoids the probability of pacing the heart during the fibrillation vulnerable period, minimizes hemodynamic deficiencies and saves battery by pacing only when necessary. However, as with asynchronous pacing, the pacing rate is not dependent on exercise and the oxygenation needs of the body.

Single and dual chamber pacemakers

Up to now we have referred to *single chamber* pacemakers, i.e. pacemakers capable of sensing and stimulating only one chamber of the heart. Early in the development of cardiac pacing [GED90], it was found that in patients where the problem was the atria to ventricles communication of the excitation (total AV block), the atria and the natural pacemaker were still working properly, modulated by physiological needs for cardiac output. In these cases it is appropriate to apply a *dual chamber* pacemaker. These pacemakers are capable of sensing both the atria and the ventricle and stimulating one or both of them depending on the pathology. Nevertheless, in many individuals the occurrence of sinus node dysfunction limits the use of atrial sensing for rate adaptation. For these last cases, *rate-adaptive pacing* has been devised. In this method the base rate of pacing is influenced by events occurring outside the heart.

Rate-adaptive pacing

The selection of a suitable method for sensing a proper indicator and adapting the heart rate accordingly must take into account the extra power consumption it involves and the need for additional sensors or leads at the outside of the pacemaker, which make implantation more complex. The main methods currently applied for adapting the heart rate ([WEB951]) do not require extra elements at the outside of the pacemaker case. They are: (1) estimating the minute ventilation (volume of air inhaled per unit of time, which has been found to be a good estimator of metabolic rate) based on the impedance of the chest, which is measured between the pacemaker case and the usual pacemaker pacing and sensing leads and (2) the measurement of body motion, mainly through an accelerometer mounted inside the pacemaker case.

None of these two approaches is perfect. Adaptation based on minute ventilation suffers from the following drawbacks. Impedance measurement tends to consume more power than efficient accelerometer circuits, and it might be affected by motion artifacts of leads and by upper body and arm swinging. In addition, it is slow to respond and it would respond to changes in respiration, like those occurring when talking during exercise or holding breath, by slowing the heart rate. On the other hand, motion sensors only track changes due to exercise and not other physiological changes that might require heart rate increase (anxiety, fever). Also in some cases they might not be able to correctly track the needs of certain exercises. This is the case of going down and going up stairs, in which, depending on the sensor and signal processing, the result might be deceptively similar in both cases or even the opposite to what is needed. In some recent pacemaker models both methods have been applied to improve adaptation.

Several other approaches have been investigated and some of them actually applied. Initially, motion based methods applied a sensor mounted on the inside wall of the case, which measured the pressure changes in the case itself. Some indicators were derived from the waveform of the intracardiac electrogram (bioelectrical signal pick up at the pacemaker leads). The measurement of changes in the blood temperature inside the veins, measured through a thermistor mounted in the pacemaker lead, was also applied.

Other functions

In the previous description of pacemakers the following functions were identified: *generation of stimulation pulses* to the heart, *sensing of the spontaneous heart activity, sensing of an indicator for heart rate adaptation* and a *processing unit* to take decisions. These functions are depicted in Figure 1-2 together with the following additional features that are included in current pacemakers.

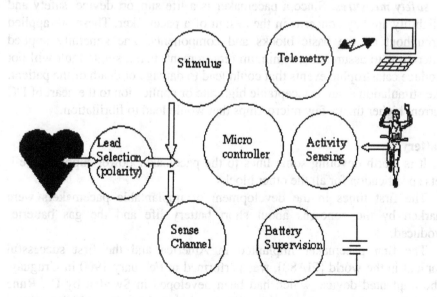

Figure 1-2. Main functions of present implantable pacemakers.

lead or polarity selection. For stimulation and sensing two electrical connections are required, let us call them the active electrode and the reference electrode. The active electrode is always at the tip of the lead, in contact with the inside wall of the heart chamber. The reference electrode can be the pacemaker case (unipolar stimulation or sensing) or a ring electrode, which is placed on the lead, 2 to 3 cm. from the tip where the active electrode is (bipolar stimulation or sensing). Then bipolar leads have two built-in conductors. Current cardiac pacemakers may be configured independently for either unipolar or bipolar stimulation or sensing. This requires a set of switches to change the connection of at least the reference connection of the sense channel and the stimulation. These switches are called lead or polarity selection block.

measurement of the battery voltage. This function detects when the battery is near depletion.

communication (telemetry). The capability to communicate with the outside of the body makes it possible to receive parameters of operation that are programmed to suit each patient (amplitude, duration and basic rate of stimulation pulses, polarity for stimulation and sensing, threshold of detection of spontaneous events, alternatives on the control algorithm of the pacemaker), and to transmit from the pacemaker statistical data of operation (number of stimuli, number of sensed events), the state of the battery, the impedance seen at the electrodes, the programmed parameters and the unit identification.

safety measures. Since a pacemaker is a life support device, safety and reliability are key concerns in the design of a pacemaker. These are applied throughout all the basic blocks and components. The generally applied criterion is to assure, as a minimum requirement, that a single fault will not produce catastrophic events that could lead to damage or death of the patient, like stimulation at an unacceptable high rate or application to the heart of DC current higher than a few microAmps that would lead to fibrillation.

Battery

It is worth devoting some lines to the pacemaker power supply since it sets specification for all the other blocks.

The first times in the development of implantable pacemakers were marked by the concerns about short battery life and the gas batteries produced.

The first pacemaker implanted in America and the first successful implant in the world [FIA88], was performed in February 1960 in Uruguay. The implanted device, which had been developed in Sweden by Dr. Rune Elmqvist, used two rechargeable nickel-cadmium batteries, which required charging through an inductive link for 12 hours about once a week. The unit implanted some months later in the USA, developed by Wilson Greatbatch, was energized by 10 mercury zinc cells ([GED90], [ADA95]). Even nuclear powered pacemakers were applied during some time, but several safety concerns were associated with them. The qualitative leap and final solution came with the introduction by Greatbatch et al. of the *lithium battery* in 1971 ([GED90]). Since 1972, lithium batteries have been used. The *lithium-iodine (Li/I₂)* battery has been the standard in the implantable cardiac pacemaker industry for over 20 years ([SAN96]).

The lithium-iodine battery yields an open circuit voltage of 2.8V. Typical internal resistance at beginning of life condition is around a few hundred ohms (100Ω to 500Ω). As the battery depletes it can be modeled with an approximately constant open circuit voltage and with a changing internal resistance that reaches several thousands ohms near depletion. The 1kHz internal AC impedance follows the same behavior. Typical evolution of output voltage and 1kHz internal AC impedance as a function of percentage of nominal charge delivered to a 100kΩ load are shown in Figure 1-3.

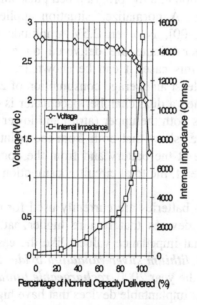

Figure 1-3. Evolution of output voltage and internal impedance for a lithium-iodine battery for 100kΩs constant resistive discharge.

From these curves stems the need for operation of pacemaker circuit blocks down-to power supply voltages of around 2V. As the voltage discharge characteristic rapidly falls near depletion, the circuit must be able to operate at this low supply voltage in order to guarantee operation during an acceptable time from the detection of the battery low condition to its replacement. The high internal impedance of the battery near the end of life also imposes the use of a considerable decoupling capacitor at the battery input lines (several tens of microFarads) to accommodate transient peaks of consumption while avoiding high amplitude glitches in the voltage supply that might mainly affect digital circuits. This situation also sets limits for the allowable current consumption peaks due to stimulation current, stimulation capacitor charging and consumption of blocks, like the communication circuit, that are seldom turned on for long times, but when they are, they may risk decreasing dangerously the supply voltage.

Implantable grade lithium-iodine batteries are available in capacities ranging from about half an Ah to a couple of Ah ([GRE03]). A representative value, for present pacemakers that tend to favor size reduction over device lifetime, might be 1Ah. This is equivalent to 114 μA year. Consequently, in order to have a 10 year lifetime for the device a total average consumption of 11.4μA is required. On the other hand, how much energy is required for stimulating the heart? This is dependent on how often the heart requires stimulation and the programmed pulse amplitude, which is adjusted for each patient. A normalized situation applied for estimating pacemaker lifetime [CEN00], is when 2.5V amplitude pulses of 0.5ms duration at 72 pulses per minute are delivered on a leads plus tissue impedance of 500Ω. In this case, it can be shown that in typical output circuit configurations, at least an average consumption of 2.8μA is required. This value is doubled when a dual chamber pacemaker is considered, i.e. a pacemaker that stimulates both the upper (atria) and lower (ventricles) parts of the heart. These figures show that both from the point of view of how much energy is available at the battery and from the comparison with the energy delivered to the heart, the total circuit consumption must be within a few microAmps.

Other types of lithium batteries are currently used for other implantable devices ([GRE03]). For devices that require higher battery currents and hence much lower internal impedance values, like the case of implantable defibrillators ([WAR96]), *lithium silver vanadium oxide (Li/SVO)* batteries have been developed. In the year 2000, *rechargeable lithium batteries* have been introduced aiming at implantable devices that have higher consumption and that would have unacceptable short lifetime with conventional lithium batteries. Examples of these devices are neurological devices, left ventricular assist devices, artificial hearts and advanced implantable hearing devices.

Finally, also in the last few years, *lithium carbon monofluoride (Li/CFx)* batteries have been introduced. They are characterized by a relatively flat voltage discharge profile, much lower internal impedance throughout its entire life and higher current capacity than lithium-iodine counterparts plus low overall cell weight. This eases circuit design, alleviating the above-mentioned restriction imposed on peak current consumption by lithium iodine batteries. Li/CFx batteries are finding their way into pacemaker, implantable defibrillators (AICD), implantable drug infusion pumps, and neurostimulator applications.

This brief overview of the pacemaker operation and functions has emphasized those aspects related to our main goal – circuit design. Before entering into the discussion of the specifications and challenges of circuit design, it is worth mentioning several other brilliant achievements in pacemaker technology. They have been accomplished in the case itself, in leads and electrodes as well as in the medical technology of implant. The pacemaker engineering and medical community has been able to solve several key issues in these areas. The following are some examples.

The biocompatibility of case, leads and electrodes and long term reliable operation in the body medium and simple implant techniques. This has lead nowadays to use, as standard packaging technique for pacemakers, a hermetically sealed titanium case. This case is filled with helium, which provides an inert, non corrosive ambient for the circuits and allows to easily detect very small leaks in the case that would lead to body fluids entering in contact with the circuitry.

Implant techniques that allow to place the pacemaker case close to the skin and take the leads through a vein towards the inside of the heart, have resulted in a rapid and secure surgical procedure.

Leads material and construction characteristics and electrode fixation techniques that reliably withstand the placement inside the permanently moving heart, with hundreds of millions of contractions in the pacemaker lifetime, while at the same time they do not produce harm or discomfort to the patient.

Figure 1-4 shows an actual pacemaker with its lead.

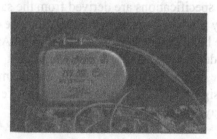

Figure 1-4. Pacemaker manufactured by CCC del Uruguay S.A. ([CCC03]), showing the titanium case and the epoxy "neck" where leads are connected.

2.   SPECIFICATIONS OF PACEMAKER CIRCUIT BLOCKS

Among the circuit blocks of a cardiac pacemaker, three broad categories can be distinguished regarding their nature: (1) the processing unit or microcontroller, (2) analog signal processing and other analog circuits (including digital auxiliary logic) and (3) the output circuits (voltage multipliers and polarity switches). In the first category we deal with pure digital circuits, in the second category with traditional analog circuits (amplifiers, filters, comparators, A/D and D/A converters) and the third category is mainly based on switches, so the involved techniques and considerations are clearly different from the other two groups. In this work we focus on the second category. In the first part of this section detailed specifications are provided on two such blocks: the sense channel and the rate adaptation sensor. Then some brief information will be provided on the third category and other analog blocks. In the final part of this section the prior published work is reviewed.

2.1   General specifications

We first consider specifications that apply to all circuit blocks.

Two general specifications are derived from the characteristics of lithium iodine batteries:
– operation from 2.8V down to at least 2V,
– current consumption of a block must be set keeping in mind the effect on the power supply voltage at the end of life condition, due to increased battery internal resistance, as well as the contribution of the block to the average consumption of the device, which determines the operating life.

Additional global specifications are derived from the safety requirements.
– No single fault may produce catastrophic events like the conduction of DC current through the heart higher than a couple of microAmps or stimulation pulses delivered at an excessively high rate.
– The fact that we are designing a high reliability device must be kept in mind during all design stages. This concerns aspects like process selection, device sizing and layout rules.

2.2   Sense Channel

The circuit that processes the bioelectric signals from the cardiac muscle to detect spontaneous cardiac activity is known as sense amplifier or sensing channel.

A standard test waveform representing the cardiac signal to be detected is the triangular wave with 2ms rise time and 13ms fall time shown in Figure 1-5 [CEN00].

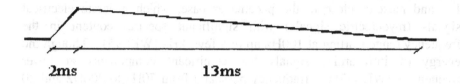

2ms   **13ms**

Figure 1-5. Standard input test signal for sense channel.

Typical thresholds of detection are amplitudes from 0.2mV to 3.2mV in the atrium and 0.4mV to 6.4mV in the ventricle in 16 programmable steps. The threshold of detection must be programmable to adapt the operation to the characteristics of each patient. The detection of these small signal amplitudes requires amplification and filtering in order to separate the desired signal from interfering signals and to reach signal amplitudes that could be reliably compared with the desired threshold. Figure 1-6 shows the basic block diagram of a sense channel.

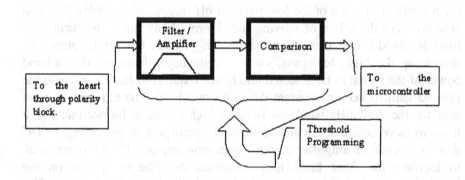

Figure 1-6. Basic block diagram of sense channel.

We will now discuss the main specifications of the filtering, amplification and comparison functions. Further characteristics of the circuit elements of the blocks, which depend on decisions concerning the overall architecture, will be discussed in Chapter 2 when the implementation details are described.

Filter / amplifier block

There are two main sources of interfering signals that are close to the frequency range of cardiac signals. They are the mains network, at 50 and 60 Hz, and muscles close to the pacemaker case, which generate electrical signals (myoelectric signals) with significant spectral content in the frequency range starting at 100Hz up to a few kHz [WEB951]. Though the energy of intracardiac signals has significant components at lower frequencies [WEB951], a frequency passband from 70Hz to 200Hz and 20 dB/dec roll-off on both sides has been proved, in several generations of pacemakers, to be a suitable choice that leaves these interfering sources out of the band while allowing the correct detection of physiological signals [CCC96].

The previous specifications for input signal and bandpass imply that if a signal amplitude of, for example, 88mV (which is the value used in the implementation described in the next Chapter) is required at the input of the comparator, a maximum gain of around 700 is needed in the bandpass to obtain a 0.2mV threshold of detection.

In order to consider the required precision on the frequency band limits, it must be noticed that the goals of interference rejection and correct detection can also be fulfilled with somewhat different cut off frequencies, particularly in the case of the low pass cut off frequency of 200Hz. We will now consider the effect of moving the filtering band limits. Reducing the filter bandwidth (i.e. increasing the low, high pass, cut off frequency or decreasing the high, low pass, cut off frequency), decreases the in-band power of the signal to be detected and hence requires to further increase the in-band gain to keep a constant detection threshold. The required in band gain for the 70-200Hz bandpass is fairly high (700); to further increase it leads to more complex circuits (additional amplifying stages or higher DC gain in operational amplifiers) with higher consumption. On the other hand, to increase the filter bandwidth decreases the filtering action on the interfering signals. Let us discuss which are the limits on this direction. The lower, high pass cut off frequency, cannot be much reduced as it is limited on the lower side by the need of filtering the 60Hz mains frequency and cardiac signals which are of lower frequency and do not correspond to the events that are to be sensed. The higher, low pass, cut off frequency is limited on the high side by the increase of the signal power of myoelectric signals that affect the output as the high cut off frequency is increased. Nevertheless, there is not a clear-cut limit here, since the spectral content of myoelectric signal is spread out in a wide band. Therefore, cut off frequencies up to 300Hz might still be acceptable.

The filter characteristics and precision, must take into account the following aspects:

a) the 70 to 200Hz frequency band is a typical specification and these nominal values might be altered while complying with the guidelines discussed in the previous paragraph.

b) the spread of the cut off frequencies around the selected nominal values must be such that it makes it possible to comply with the desired precision in the detection thresholds, which will be discussed below.

Based on these principles, a precision of +/- 10Hz in the low frequency cut off frequency and +/- 20 Hz in the high frequency cut off, are specified.

In addition to the sources of interfering signals previously mentioned, radio frequency signals must also be considered. These signals, though lying well above the sense filter band, may also affect the sense circuitry due to demodulation occurring in semiconductor junctions that could lead to low frequency spurious signals. Radio frequency interference is prevented from reaching the sense circuitry through the metallic enclosure of the pacemaker and through capacitors that shunt the leads to the case.

Filtering is not the only measure for interference prevention. The bipolar sensing method, mentioned in Section 1.2, where a lead with two built-in conductors brings the input signal to the pacemaker, is a measurement technique more robust than unipolar sensing, in which the pacemaker case acts as the reference electrode. In bipolar sensing the loop area sensible to electromagnetic interference is greatly reduced and interfering signals become mainly common mode signals. Nowadays pacemakers can be configured in either unipolar or bipolar sensing, the bipolar method usually being the preferred one when the lowest values of the threshold of detection are applied.

Additional requirements relate to the connection of the sense block to the pacemaker leads. The input impedance must be greater than about 20kΩ in order to avoid loading the tissues excessively and consequently affecting the measured signal. Since the sense channel and the stimulation circuit share the same connection leads to the heart, it is required that the circuit recovers from the effect of stimulating pulses (that can have amplitudes up to about 7.5V), quickly enough (in less than about 100ms in traditional pacemaker sense amplifiers). Finally, the application of the previously mentioned safety criteria influences the way this connection is made. Usually an external capacitor, which makes part of the filtering section, is included to assure that a single fault will not lead to the delivery of a dangerous DC current through the heart. An accepted safe limit for the fault condition is a DC current of 2μA.

Comparison block

Once the signal has been filtered and amplified, it is compared with a threshold level to decide whether the heart contraction occurred. Regarding comparison speed, neither the slow varying input signal nor the dynamics of the application, which evolves at "biological" speed, are much demanding. Detection delays below a couple of ms are acceptable for an input signal amplitude two times the programmed threshold [CCC96] (since the comparator delay is dependent on input overdrive).

Precision of detection thresholds

Two issues influence the requirement on the accuracy of detection thresholds.

First, there is no need for a high precision since the threshold of detection is selected for each patient at the implant time and the procedure applied to select this threshold does not depend on the accuracy of threshold levels in absolute terms. This procedure is based on checking that the device systematically detects the signal of the patient and will not detect interfering signals.

Second is the fact that the lowest threshold values are the most affected by circuits imperfections since for these thresholds the highest gain or lowest comparison levels are applied. Therefore, considering a constant accuracy specification for all the threshold levels leads to either a too stringent specification for the lowest thresholds or an excessively high error specification for the rest of the threshold levels. The first alternative imposes the application of more complex circuit techniques (e.g. offset cancellation techniques) in order to comply with the specification, thus increasing power consumption.

Taking these two aspects into account we will consider a +/-25% precision specification for the lowest thresholds and +/- 10% for the rest of the thresholds.

Consumption

The sense block must be active during most part (around 70% to 80%) of the cardiac cycle and dual chamber pacemakers require two of these circuits. Typical figures for the allowed consumption of each of these blocks are around 1μA, as in reference [LEN01]. This accounts for 10 to 20 % of the total pacemaker consumption.

Recent trends on sense channel requirements

Finally, some comments on recent trends of sense channel requirements are pertinent here.

A recent improvement in pacemakers is the capture verification feature [RIT98]. This feature is based on detecting whether a stimulation pulse has been effective by sensing the cardiac signal very rapidly (between 15 to 45 ms) after the stimulation pulse (a technique referred to as "early sensing"). In this way the stimulation amplitude can be adapted to the minimum required, which saves energy. Currently, the stimulation pulse amplitude is fixed for each patient at the implant time according to what is measured. In this case, after stimulation (or spontaneous contraction) there is a "refractory" period of about 15 to 30% of the cardiac cycle, where the cardiac signal is not sensed.

This feature involves modifications at the electrode, input interface of the sense channel and filtering, in order to avoid the transient perturbations due to the stimulus. In reference [LEN01] a bandpass filter with 40dB/dec high pass and 20dB/dec low pass characteristics is applied, and measures are included to discharge the filter capacitors and to change the compensation of the input amplifier in order to speed up the circuit response during the early sensing phase, after the stimulus pulse. In our design we will not include this feature. However, the data from reference [LEN01], shows that the modifications in the filtering stage are small (basically a 2nd order high pass section instead of a first order high pass section). Hence, our conclusions can be extended to this case.

Another trend is to include the capability of acquiring, storing and transmitting short sequences of the input signal to the sense channel (intracardiac electrogram) for diagnostic purposes. This information is also used in some models to measure the actual amplitude of the incoming signal and automatically adjust the detection threshold [GUI03].

Table 1-1 summarizes the sense channel specifications.

Table 1-1. Specifications summary of sense channel.

Specification	Required value
Supply voltage	2.0 –2.8V
Total current consumption	< 1µA
Frequency response	Bandpass, 70- 200Hz, first order high and low pass.
Input amplitude thresholds (CENELEC Test signal [CEN00])	0.2mV to 3.2mV in the atrium, 0.4mV to 6.4mV in the ventricle in 16 programmable steps.
Required maximum in-band gain	700 for 88mV output at 0.2mV input.
Threshold accuracy	+/-25% of nominal value (lowest values) +/-10% of nominal value (highest values)

Specification	Required value
Detection delay	< 2ms for input signal amplitude equal to twice the programmed threshold.
Input Impedance	> 20kΩ
Safety	DC current through input leads < 2µA for single fault condition.

2.3   Rate Adaptation Sensor

Several approaches exist, as noted above, for sensing a magnitude suitable for rate adaptation. We will limit ourselves to the case of sensing acceleration. The specifications are those of the industrial circuit we developed ([ARN98]).

The range of accelerations, appearing at chest level due to normal human exercise, ranges approximately from 0.007g to 0.34g. At the lower limit of 0.007g the available signal in the usual sensors is in the few µV region, hence requiring paying particular attention to the noise characteristics of the circuits involved. The frequency band of interest was fixed at 0.5Hz to 7Hz, which also corresponds to what is reported in [WEB951] for several studies on acceleration characteristics for various activities. First order high pass and low pass characteristics were deemed sufficient. As an indicator of the average exertion level, the circuit must deliver at its output the average of the absolute value of the acceleration during three seconds. The absolute value is considered because both acceleration and de-accelerations are significant. The current consumption budget allowed to this module was 3µA.

Figure 1-7 shows the basic block diagram of a rate adaptation sensor and Table 1-2 summarizes its specifications.

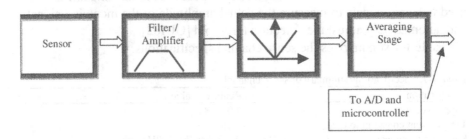

Figure 1-7. Basic block diagram of acceleration based rate adaptation sensor.

Piezoelectric, piezoresistive and capacitive sensors have been applied to acceleration sensing in pacemakers. In our case the targeted sensor was a piezoresistive sensor. Piezoresistive sensors present some advantages. They are available in discrete form and their cost is much smaller than piezoelectric sensors which are the other ones also available in discrete form. In addition they are suitable for integration in silicon through micromachining techniques. Despite these benefits, their resistive nature and resistance value, usually in the $K\Omega$ range ([WEB951],[ICS00]), impair the application in a micropower environment. Appendix 2 presents the technique we applied to overcome this limitation.

Table 1-2. Specifications summary for rate adaptation sensor.

Specification	Required value
Supply voltage	2.0 –2.8V
Total current consumption	< 3µA
Frequency response	Bandpass, 0.5- 7Hz, first order high and low pass.
Input amplitudes	0.007g to 0.34g

2.4 Other Analog Blocks

Further analog circuits are used in a pacemaker.

An A/D converter is required for measuring the output of the rate adaptation circuit and battery voltage measurement. A precision of eight bits is usually enough and this block is sometimes a standard peripheral block of the microcontroller device or core.

The telemetry function calls for analog functions, particularly in the receiver section. In our case, where the inbound communication to the pacemaker applies On-Off-Keying (OOK) modulation, a comparator based receiver can be applied ([BAR98]). The speed requirements are higher than in the sense channel case, since the incoming signals are usually in the kHz range. The allowed consumption is also higher and it can be up to tens of µA, but only during short periods.

For the battery voltage measurement function, besides the A/D converter a voltage reference is needed. In this case, the current consumption requirement is also relaxed because the block is on only once each cardiac cycle, during the very short period needed to take the measurement.

Finally a special reference current source is needed for biasing the circuits in the nA range ([VIT77], [VIT93]).

2.5 Pulse Generation

All pacemakers nowadays apply a capacitor discharge, quasi-constant voltage pulse for stimulation. Basically a capacitor charged to a preprogrammed voltage ("tank" capacitor, C_{tank}) is connected to the heart during a given time.

When higher amplitude pulses are required the tank capacitor can be connected in series with the power supply.

The connection of the tank capacitor to the heart is usually done through a discharged series capacitor (C_{series}). This series capacitor, though decreasing the effective stimulation capacitance, helps in two ways: (1) it assures the safety condition that no single fault can lead to the delivery of a DC current to the heart and (2) when it is discharged through the heart after the pulse, it nulls the total charge delivered to the heart. This effect of nulling the total charge delivered to the heart helps in alleviating the phenomenon of "electrode polarization" or "afterpotentials" ([WEB951]) that refer to the potentials appearing at the leads due to the charges accumulated in the electrode-tissue interface due to the stimulation pulse. These afterpotentials might later mask the heart signals that need to be sensed.

Modern pacemakers are capable of delivering programmable pulses with amplitudes that range from about 0.2V to around 7.0V, with widths from 0.1ms up to 2ms. This means generating voltages from one tenth to 3 times the battery voltage. The values of the series and tank capacitors required to reach stimulation are in the 10 to 30μF range and therefore are always external components. The typical impedance seen due to the combination of leads, electrode-tissue interface and tissues is about 500Ω, the expected values being from 400Ω to 1000Ω. This calls for very low on-resistance switches, since the circuit and some of the switches must then handle currents up to 14 mA, i.e. around 7V over 500Ω, with low voltage fall (less than 100mV).

Figure 1-8 depicts a simplified diagram of a pacemaker output stage corresponding to one of the chambers of the heart during the charge and stimulation phases. The terminals S+ and S- represent the bipolar terminals that are inside one heart chamber (A+ and A- for the atrium and V+ and V- for the ventricle in a dual chamber pacemaker). The CASE terminal is connected to the pacemaker case. The switches S_{CASE} and S_{S+}, which are part of the polarity block, allow to select between unipolar stimulation (referred to the pacemaker case) and bipolar stimulation (referred to the ring electrode S+ in a bipolar lead).

In summary, the main challenges posed by the design of the output circuit are: (1) the need for high current, low resistance switches; (2) the requirement of handling voltages outside the power supply range that demands specialized techniques for turning on and off the switches and makes more complex the issues of on chip protections and latch-up prevention, and (3) the management of these aspects in a low-power supply voltage environment with very low overhead current drains (clearly below 1μA).

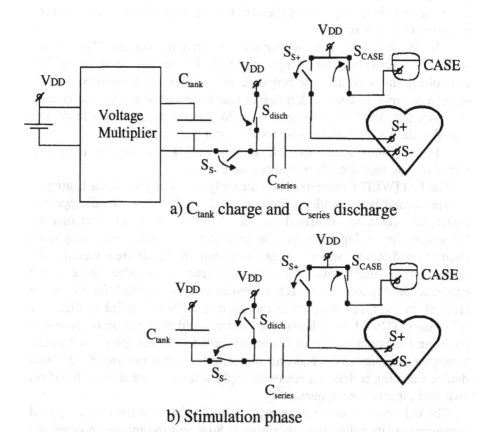

a) C_{tank} charge and C_{series} discharge

b) Stimulation phase

Figure 1-8. Simplified diagram of charge and stimulation phases of pacemaker output stage corresponding to one chamber of the heart. Stimulation polarity is selected by keeping closed either S_{S+} (bipolar stimulation) or S_{CASE} (unipolar stimulation). During the charging of the tank capacitor and discharging of the series capacitor, S_{S-} is open and S_{disch} is closed. For stimulation, the tank capacitor is disconnected from the voltage multiplier, S_{disch} is opened and S_{S-} is closed.

2.6   Prior published works

As noted in the preface of [WEB951], little information is available in the open technical literature regarding the design details of cardiac pacemaker circuits and even less for integrated circuits. This is probably due to the "closed" characteristic of the pacemaker industry (few companies with a long tradition) and the high competition among these companies. Many architectural design details are included in the thousands of patents in the field. However, when circuit design details are dealt with in the case of patents, which is not the most common case, actual performance results are not presented since they are not relevant for the claim of innovation purpose of a patent description.

In the following lines we summarize what is available. This is one source of information for comparison with the results achieved in SOI technology and with the new proposed architectures. Additionally we will refer to our own industrial chip design that is described in the next chapter and prior published work on general analog circuit design issues (amplifier and filter design) that will be discussed in later chapters.

From bibliographic research among leading journals on integrated circuit design, four specific references were found.

The first [WEI70] corresponds to the early stages of pacemaker history.

The second is the work by Stotts et al [STO892], from the disappeared pacemaker company Intermedics, on a custom chip for pacemakers. Regarding the analog circuitry, the chip did not include rate adaptation circuitry, and though an interesting discussion on the different methods for implementing filters with high time constants is included, there is no complete description of the actual implementation applied for the sense channel. In the block diagram of the sense amplifier included as Fig. 5 of reference [STO892], it is shown that the threshold of detection is controlled by using the variable gain of the amplifier/filter, whose gain is selectable through a capacitor array. This and another reference to the use of correlated double sampling techniques seems to imply that the sense stage is based on switched capacitor techniques.

The only data given on consumption establishes that the overall typical consumption (including the processor) is 8μA and the minimum operating voltage 1.7V.

The third and fourth papers ([NOV99] and [NOV01]) present the design of an output stage.

Regarding conference proceedings, presentations have recently come from Italian groups, mainly related to the University of Padova and the pacemaker company Medico ([LEN01], [GER011], [GER00], [GER012], [BAS01]).

In Reference [LEN01], Lentola et al. describe the implementation of an atrial sensing channel in a 0.8μm Bulk CMOS technology. The circuit is based on two external 47nF decoupling capacitors, a continuous time differential preamplifier, a third order (1st order high-pass cascaded with 2nd order band-pass) switched capacitor filter, 5 bits DAC for threshold voltage programmability and comparator. The proposed filtering is suitable for "early sensing" applications. The total consumption is 1μA (of these 0.45μA are drawn by the preamplifier and 0.15μA by the switched capacitor filter) and minimum operating voltage is 2V. The noise amplitude is 5.1mVrms at the filter output.

Gerosa et al, propose in [GER011], a class AB log-domain 2nd order band-pass filter / amplifier, in 0.8µm Bulk CMOS technology. The amplifier provides a programmable gain from 50dB to 70dB. This filter has no automatic tuning and is intended to provide rough filtering, with the required pass-band fixed by a following stage. The log-domain amplifier dissipates 2.8 µW, i.e. also 1µA at 2.8V, not including the comparator and following filtering stages. This amplifier presents 1.7µVrms noise at the input.

The alternatives for the following filtering stages after this log-domain amplifier are presented by the same authors in references [GER00] and [GER012]. In [GER00] they propose an architecture for the acquisition and digitization of cardiac signals in a pacemaker, based on Sigma-Delta modulation. Then further filtering would be provided in the digital domain. According to simulations the dynamic range achieved by this Sigma-Delta modulator is larger than 50dB with an oversampled frequency of 8kHz.

In reference [GER012] they compare this solution with a switched capacitor (SC) band-pass filtering solution. The circuits, implemented in 0.8µm CMOS technology, can operate at a minimum voltage of 2V while consuming, including the preceding log-domain amplifier, 5µW (i.e. 1.8µA @ 2.8V) for the Sigma-Delta modulator solution and 3.6µW (i.e. 1.3µA @ 2.8V) for the SC solution. When analyzing and comparing these results it must be pointed out that, on the one hand, the power consumption in the Sigma-Delta case seems only to include the modulator and not the following digital signal processing stages and, on the other hand, in references [GER011],[GER00] and [GER012] the results provided come only from simulations.

Finally, a 4th order bandpass switched-opamp switched capacitor filter based on the switched-opamp technique for sense channel application is presented by Baschirotto et al in [BAS01]. It operates from a 1V power supply, consuming 1.2µW. Sampling frequency is 1kHz and is implemented in 0.35µm standard CMOS technology. Though the low supply voltage achieved is an interesting feature, nevertheless this is not the case in actual pacemaker circuits.

These results show that the current consumption reached in published work is at least 1µA.

Let us conclude this description of the specification of cardiac pacemakers circuits by pointing out that, though the trend of expanding pacemaker features has been possible due to the evolution of microelectronic systems, the reduction of power consumption (to increase the device lifetime) and size (which is linked to consumption through the battery size) are still central goals [SAN96]. Our work addresses this challenge for the case of the analog circuitry through the joint application of SOI technology and novel design approaches.

3.   OTHER MEDICAL DEVICES

This section reviews the basic specifications of other medical functions and devices. The comparison of these specifications with those of cardiac pacemakers will allow us to analyze the scope of application of the result of this work.

Our work centers on analog signal processing functions that are associated to measurement blocks of pacemakers. Several other measurements are of interest in the medical domain. Table 1-3 summarizes the main characteristics of various examples. They are classified according to whether they are of interest for present or future implantable devices or they correspond to techniques applied in external devices.

Implantable devices generally require the measurement of physiological parameters in order to operate in a closed loop. This is the case in pacemakers and is also the case of Functional Electrical Stimulation (FES) systems mentioned in the Table. FES systems aim at artificially restoring bodily functions, such a those provided by an organ or limb, particularly in cases where is missing the normal brain command through the neural system, e.g. when a spinal cord injury exists. The first part of the Table summarizes this kind of feedback measurements that are related to implantable devices. Along with this feedback purpose, there exist measurements which are interesting even separate from stimulation capabilities. This is the case of monitoring of glucose concentration in blood ([HEL99], [SHU94]).

The second part of the table presents examples of measurements taken from the surface of the body and thus applied in external devices.

A common characteristic of medical measurements is variability. As stated in [WEB952]: "Most measured quantities vary with time, even when all controllable factors are fixed. Many medical measurements vary widely among normal patients, even when conditions are similar". Therefore, in most of cases, it does not make sense to perform high precision measurements; rather medium to low precision and signal to noise ratio are enough, particularly for providing a qualitative feedback for stimulation systems.

When we compare the signal characteristics (amplitude, frequency) to what was presented in the case of the pacemaker sense channel (which corresponds to the first row of the table), it appears the similitude with the other cases presented. A broader range of agreement results if we compare to both the sense channel and the accelerometer circuit, which reaches lower amplitude and frequency values. Nevertheless, two main differences are noted. First, the requirement of measuring the DC component in some systems, which would impose the application of offset cancelling techniques. Second, the fact that neural and myoelectric signals extend to higher frequencies, whose main impact would be on the consumption achievable. The consumption issue is further discussed below.

Table 1-3. Basic specifications of medical and physiological measurements.

Parameter or measuring technique	Frequency Range (Hz)	Amplitude Range (Note 1)	Intended Application
With current or foreseen application in implantable devices			
Intra-cavital ElectroCardioGram (ECG)	30 ... 200	0.1 ... 10 mV	Cardiac Implantable Devices (Pacemakers, Defibrillators, Ventricular Assist Devices)
Acceleration	0.5 ... 10	0.01 ... 1 mV	Pacemakers
Nerve potentials	DC ... 10000	0.01 ... 1 mV	Functional Electrical Stimulation (FES)
Myoelectric signals (signals from muscles)	DC ... 10000	0.1 ... 5mV	Functional Electrical Stimulation (FES)
Biochemical Sensors, (particularly for Glucose)	DC ... 0.1	nA [SHU94, LAM92]	Diabetes Management
Pressure Sensors	DC ... 50	10μV... 10mV	Blood [PAR98] and Bladder Pressure Monitoring
Applied in external devices			
Surface ElectroCardioGram (ECG)	0.01 ... 250	0.5 ... 4mV	Monitoring, from skin electrodes
ElectroEncephaloGram (EEG)	DC ... 150	0.005 ... 0.3 mV	Monitoring, from scalp electrodes

Source: [WEB952], except those related to pacemakers and where otherwise noted.
Note 1. Representative values of sensor voltage or current output are indicated when the measured magnitude is not directly a voltage.

The measurements that are aimed at implantable devices have similar constraints to the acceptable consumption levels as pacemakers. This is hard to achieve in cases where higher frequencies and lower amplitudes, and hence lower noise, are sought, as in some cases where neural signals are involved. The requirement on consumption in devices that deal with the neural system is often further strained by the need for having several measurement channels. In these cases, the solution has been the application of RF powered implants [AKI98]. The recently announced rechargeable implantable grade batteries (see Section 1.2) could provide an alternative solution. Powering the implant by RF energy allows to operate with much higher consumption levels. Nevertheless, to save power is still a concern, in order to improve the size, weight and autonomy of the external device that powers the implant and to expand the capabilities of the implant, while respecting the safety limits for energy transfer through the skin and tissues.

Finally, power is also a concern in external devices for monitoring, since portability is sometimes a desirable feature, as in the case of cardiac Holter studies.

The advance of microtechnologies and medical research makes possible new medical devices to reach the market and originates a larger number of feasibility studies and prototype development efforts. This trend is particularly intense in the case of implantable devices. In the implantable area new medical methods are devised (e.g. Parkinson's disease treatment through neurostimulation at the brain [BRA98] or evolution of pacemakers aimed at treating heart failure (heart pumping deficiency) [MOO01]) and existing functions are transferred to implantable form to improve performance or patient comfort (e.g. glucose sensors [HEL99]). Along with devices intended for clinical application, we have those aimed at aiding biomedical research, as the project presented in [PAR98], where we contributed to the development of an implantable telemetry unit aimed at biomedical research applications.

The systematization in this book of novel techniques and design methods aimed at low power design of analog circuits, together with the application of SOI technology, is believed to be a tool for aiding in solving the challenges presented by these new generations of medical devices.

4.   CONCLUSIONS

The operation of cardiac pacemakers and the constraints and specifications of its blocks have been presented.

The essential characteristics of the sense channel, which will be the main research example for this book, may be summarized as follows:

Low frequency, low order band-pass filtering with high (700) in-band gain is required.

Intended for qualitative signal detection, thus medium signal to noise ratio (40dB) is enough.

Consumption below 1μA and operation with 2V power supply are needed.

These characteristics are also required in many others medical measurement functions, particularly those included in implantable devices. The advances in microtechnologies are giving birth to new devices that will benefit from the improvements achieved in the fulfillment of these characteristics.

Chapter 2

Industrial Implementation of Pacemaker Integrated Circuit in Bulk CMOS Technology

This chapter will discuss the architectural alternatives, trade-offs, actual design and results of circuits we have implemented in Bulk CMOS technology, for a pacemaker's analog processing functions.

The analysis of this industrial design will provide us with detailed specifications and performance data that will be later applied to design and evaluate alternative architectures and technology (SOI).

Particularly, we will focus on the sense channel design, which is the main example of application circuit considered in this book. In addition, the design of the activity sense block is described in Appendix 2. The design of this last block further exemplifies the techniques applied to achieve micropower consumption and correct operation at 2V power supply in a standard Bulk technology.

The designs are part of the ASIC for implantable cardiac pacemakers developed at the Instituto de Ingeniería Eléctrica, Universidad de la República, Uruguay, under a contract with the Centro de Construcción de Cardioestimuladores del Uruguay S.A. [CCC03]. The ASIC includes all the circuitry of a dual chamber implantable pacemaker except for the microcontroller: sense channels, signal conditioning and processing circuitry for an accelerometer for rate adaptation, programmable voltage multipliers for stimulation, polarity switches, battery voltage supervision, demodulation for short range telemetry, microprocessor interface and current reference. It occupies a die area of $36mm^2$ in a standard 2.4μm analog CMOS process with double poly and double metal. This process is intended for 5V power supply and has nominal threshold voltages of nMOS (pMOS) transistors of 0.85V (-0.85V) with minimum and maximum specified values of, respectively, 0.7V (-0.7V) and 1.0V (-1.0V). The fulfillment of the 2V requirement in such a process, presents challenges due to the detrimental effect of low supply voltage on aspects like analog switches on-resistance, operational amplifier input common mode range and output swing, which will be further discussed in the following chapter. The methods required to overcome these limitations are considered in this chapter for the case of the sense channel and in Appendix 2 for the accelerometer signal conditioning circuit.

Some results derived from the work developed in this project are included in publications [BAR96],[ARN98],[ARN97] and [BAR98].

Figure 2-1 shows a photograph of a production chip. The project is in industrial phase. The chip is being produced in volume (yield of 81%) after passing qualification (reliability assessment) tests [EUR01].

The layout of the circuit is shown in Figure 2-2.

The rest of the chapter discusses the design of the sense channel. The selection of the overall architecture and the main design characteristics of the basic building blocks are presented. In particular the compromise involved between the use of external components and the implementation of fully integrated solutions is discussed.

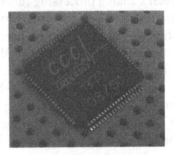

Figure 2-1. Photograph of production chip of ASIC for pacemakers.

1.   SENSE CHANNEL DESIGN

As described in the previous chapter, the implementation of the sense channel requires amplification / filtering and comparison to detect a programmable amplitude of the input signal. Concerning the overall architecture, the main alternatives in order to implement this programmable threshold of detection are to have a variable gain amplifier and a fixed comparison threshold or a fixed gain amplifier with a variable comparison threshold or a combination of both. We selected the second alternative, whose basic block diagram is shown in Figure 2-3.

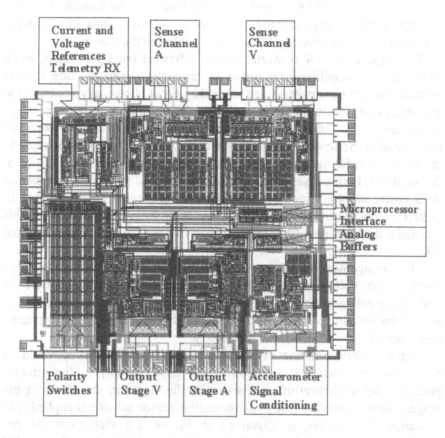

Figure 2-2. Layout of Bulk CMOS industrial ASIC for pacemakers. This chip includes all the modules of a dual chamber pacemaker except for the microcontroller, which is a separate chip.

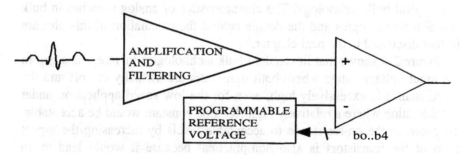

Figure 2-3. Basic sense channel architecture.

As described in [BAR96] and explained hereafter, the variable threshold is appropriately implemented through a classic capacitive charge redistribution D/A converter [MCC75] for the following reasons.

This capacitive D/A converter can be refreshed once per cardiac cycle while the sense amplifier is not active. In this capacitive architecture, there is no static current consumption and since the output is basically constant, the dynamic power consumption is negligible. To have 16 programming steps for the sensitivity of the circuit, the central 16 levels of a 5 bits D/A with full scale equal to the supply voltage can be used. This avoids operation close to the supply rails for the input stage of the comparator and the output stage of the amplifier. In this case, each threshold step at the input of the comparator is the power supply divided by 32; i.e. 87.5mV at nominal supply voltage. In order to allow detection of input test signals of 0.2mV amplitude with this threshold, the band-pass filter must have an in-band maximum gain of about 700.

This arrangement introduces a dependency of the threshold of detection on the supply voltage corresponding to a variation by 28% near end of life (2V supply voltage). Better results can be achieved if a bandgap reference is applied for the D/A converter. This of course has the drawback of increased consumption.

The alternative solution involving a variable gain amplifier would be more complex since the operation at 2V power supply in this process precludes the utilization of switches to handle signal in the whole supply range, unless an on-chip clock voltage-multiplication scheme is applied. The limitation of switches is illustrated in Figure 2-4 that plots the on-conductance and on-resistance of a switch, implemented as the parallel connection of a n and a pMOS transistor driven by complementary signals, as a function of the input voltage of the switch. This graph depicts the case of a typical bulk technology. The characteristics of analog switches in bulk and SOI technologies and the details behind the calculation of this plot are further discussed in the next chapter.

Figure 2-4 shows that in standard bulk technologies there exists a gap in the input voltage range where both transistors are virtually cut off and the on-resistance is excessively high, even for the low speed application under consideration where a relatively high RC time constant would be acceptable. To decrease the on-resistance to acceptable levels by increasing the aspect ratio of the transistors is also non-practical because it would lead to an unacceptable charge injection error.

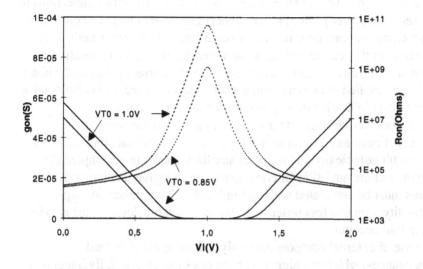

Figure 2-4. On-conductance (solid lines) and resistance (dashed lines) of Bulk CMOS switch vs. input voltage for 2V power supply with nominal threshold voltage (VT0 = 0.85V) and maximum threshold voltage (VT0 = 1.0V) for both nMOS and pMOS transistors. This plot was calculated applying the EKV model ([VIT93,ENZ95]) with a body-effect coefficient of 1.5 (see next chapter for further details).

Let us discuss the implementation alternatives and trade-offs in the amplification and filtering stage. We will first consider two aspects: the impact on the overall system of having some external components and the constraints imposed by the large time constants and high gain required.

1.1 Fully integrated vs. external components

One first issue is the fully integrated vs. external components dilemma. On this issue, the following points must be taken into account.
1. The trend of reducing size in implantable devices is very clear ([SAN96]) and easy to understand since it makes the implant more physically and psychologically comfortable for the patient. However, as we previously pointed out, we must keep in mind that the overall implant size is linked to consumption through the battery size. Therefore the fully integrated vs. external components discussion has a third party that is the resulting consumption and its impact on battery size or duration.
2. External components are practically unavoidable. In the case of the Sense Channel, they are related to the safety requirement that a single fault will

not provoke catastrophic failures like DC current higher than a very low leakage current passing through the heart. One way to guarantee this condition is to have an external capacitor in series with the connections to the sense amplifier prior to other connections. In this way, DC current is blocked by this capacitor in case of occurrence of any other fault. In case of a fault in this capacitor (e.g. a short circuit), the normal operation of the rest of the circuit guarantees there is no DC current going to the heart. This was applied in our case and a 47nF external capacitor is also applied in [LEN01] in this location, probably for the same reasons.

3. When considering fully integrated solutions, other factors must be evaluated besides consumption. These are the impact on chip size due to the circuit complexity and required auxiliary blocks (e.g. sampled data circuits require anti-alias filtering stages and integrated continuous time filters must be associated with tuning blocks). The impact on chip testability, due to a less observable and controllable device must also be taken into account.

4. The use of external components imply to handle off-chip load capacitances, which are higher than the ones required in fully integrated solutions. This might result in an increase in power consumption higher than the one due to the more complex circuitry of fully integrated solutions. However, the application of a class AB output stage, as the one proposed in Chapter 5, highly reduces the consumption penalty due to this load in quiescent conditions, which is the condition the stage is most of the time.

To summarize, we consider important and useful to search for fully integrated solutions. However, to be inflexible or obstinate on this issue may block the way to better solutions from the point of view of the global system.

1.2   Filter implementation alternatives: the large time constants and large gain problems

A second question is the actual circuit architecture. This is marked by two key specifications: filter characteristics and consumption.

We will start by considering the filter characteristics.

Our basic specification calls for a low order filter (a second order band pass filter with 20dB/dec roll-off at both sides of the band). The auxiliary blocks that are required in some circuit techniques are an overhead to this simple filter that cannot be afforded when the goal is to minimize power consumption. This is the case for the anti-alias filter in switched capacitor blocks and automatic tuning stages in integrated continuous time filters.

Other key characteristics of the filter are its low frequency (70Hz to 200Hz) and high gain (about 700).

The implementation of large time constants requires either high capacitor values or high resistor (or equivalent) or both. Let us illustrate this for the sense channel filter, considering the time constant corresponding to 70Hz, i.e. $(1/2.\Pi.70)$, which is equal to 2.3ms. The actual time constant would be a little different since 70Hz is the desired -3dB frequency that in this narrow filter will be slightly different from the filter poles, but let us apply this value as representative of the time constants involved in the filter.

We will consider the four circuit techniques shown in Figure 2-5: an active RC filter, a MOSFET-C filter, where the resistor is implemented by the linear region resistance of a MOSFET, a transconductance – C (gm-C) filter and a switched capacitor filter.

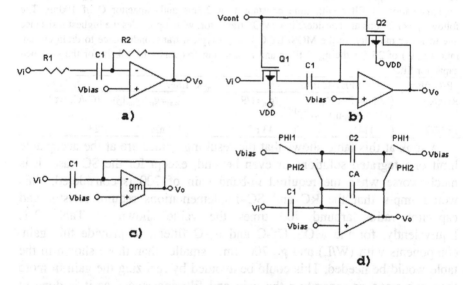

Figure 2-5. First order, high pass filtering sections considered for evaluation of feasibility of implementation of large time constants. a) Active RC, b) MOSFET-C, c) g_m-C and d) switched capacitors architectures.

An approach for implementation of filtering functions that has gained attention in the last decade, particularly for a low supply voltage environment, is log-domain filters ([ADA79], [SEE90], [FRE93], [ENZ98]). However from the point of view of the implementation of large time constants, the time constants in log-domain filters are given by $C.n.U_T/I_{bias}$, where n is the body-effect coefficient of MOS transistors, U_T is the thermal voltage and I_{bias} is the bias current of an MOS transistor operating in the weak inversion region, in order to provide the exponential characteristic required to implement log-domain filters. Considering the g_m/I_D ratio in weak inversion is a constant equal to $1/n.U_T$ (see [VIT93,ENZ95] and section 1, Chapter 3), the time constant can be rewritten as C / ($I_{bias}.(g_m/I_D$ @ weak inversion)), which is equal to C/g_m, thus leading to the same required I_{bias} as the one considered below for g_m-C filters.

If we limit the capacitance value to 100pF as a maximum value that could be integrated, then Table 2-1 shows the required value of: (1) resistance (R) for a RC filter, (2) transistor aspect ratio (W/L) for a MOSFET-C filter, (3) transconductance (g_m) and bias current required for a g_m-C filter and (4) the capacitor ratio required in a switched capacitor (SC) filter with a sampling frequency f_s of 10kHz.

The detailed calculation criteria are presented in Appendix 1.

Table 2-1. Required components characteristics for RC, MOSFET-C, g_m–C and SC implementation of filter with time constant τ of 2.3ms and capacitor C of 100pF. The following conditions are considered: a pMOS transistor, which provides the highest resistance due to lower mobility, in the MOSFET-C filter; a typical transconductance to drain current ratio (g_m/I_D) of 25 for the g_m-C filter and a sampling frequency of 10kHz for the switched capacitor filter.

R-C filter	MOSFET-C filter		g_m–C filter		SC filter
R= τ/C	(W/L)=(R.μ.C$_{ox}$. $\lvert(V_{GB}$-V_{t0}-n.$V_{SB})\rvert$)$^{-1}$	g_m=1/R	I_{bias}=g_m/(g_m/I_D)	(C$_2$/C$_1$)=τ.f$_s$	
23 MΩ	(1 / 414)	43 nS	1.7 nA	23	

A look at this table shows that the resulting values are at the acceptable limit of integrated solutions or even beyond, except for the SC case. It is much worse when the required in-band gain of 700 is considered. This would imply that the RC and SC implementations require resistor and capacitor ratios around 700 times the value shown in Table 2-1. Equivalently, for the MOSFET-C and g_m-C filters, to provide this gain, components with (W/L) and g_m 700 times smaller than those shown in the table would be needed. This could be avoided by realizing the gain in more than one stage or separating the gain and filtering stages as it is done in [LEN01] and [GER012]. However, this might lead to higher consumption, as more operational amplifiers are required, though the requirements for them would be different in both cases.

The results of Table 2-1 are based on the straightforward implementation of each filtering technique. Several efforts have been deployed for a long time to develop techniques to ease the integration of large time constants. These techniques are reviewed in Appendix 1. The analysis of these methods leads to the conclusion that though viable, their application to achieve full integration of the required large time constants and gain, must pay the price of an increased power consumption, that may derive from additional circuit functions to achieve the desired time constants (as in the case of capacitance multiplication techniques discussed in Appendix 1) or that may stem from applying an integrated filter with auxiliary functions as tuning or anti-alias filtering or increased bandwidth requirements in SC circuits. In the case of the industrial chip implementation, the greatly increased complexity was also a concern for reliability, yield and development time reasons. All these reasons lead to our decision of applying an active RC filter with external passive components, some of which are, in any case, needed for the explained safety requirements. Nevertheless, for comparison purposes, an implementation applying switched capacitor circuits was also designed and tested. It will be discussed in Chapter 6.

1.3   Final sense channel architecture

The solution we applied for the sense channel filter amplifier was a single stage one. This solution is presented in the following paragraphs in the way it is implemented in the industrial pacemaker chip. In Chapter 6 we will present a version of this architecture on Fully-Depleted SOI technology, which by taking advantage of novel amplifier design approaches, achieves a record ultra-low consumption.

The basic architecture of the filter amplifier is shown in Figure 2-6.

The bandpass filtering and amplifying function is based on the operational amplifier and external passive components R1, R2, C1 and C2. The output of the filter is compared with the programmable threshold set by the 5 bits D/A.

The CL capacitor shown at the output of the op amp represents the parasitic capacitance at this node, which is increased due to the connection of off-chip components at this node. The total loading requirements on the op amp are discussed below when the op amp specifications are considered.

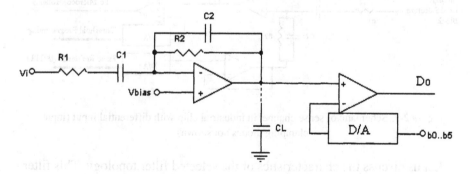

Figure 2-6. Basic sense channel amplifier / filter architecture. From [SIL021], © 2002 IEEE.

The actual circuit is completed with clamping diodes and serial switches, not shown, required to isolate the circuit from the stimulation pulses.

The Vbias voltage, which fixes the common mode voltage at the op amp input and the quiescent voltage at its output, is generated as follows. A second capacitive D/A converter, identical to the one that generates the programmable comparison threshold is used. The input to this second D/A converter is fixed at 00111, setting the quiescent level at the input and output of the amplifier at (7/32) of the supply voltage (or reference voltage of the D/A converters). This method allows precise tracking between the quiescent output level and the programmable threshold. The only drawback is larger die area. The selected quiescent level of (7/32) of the power supply voltage suits the input common mode range and output swing of the amplifier and the input range of the comparator. This quiescent level, displaced towards ground, is coherent with the input signal, which is a negative pulse that generates a positive pulse at the output of the amplifier. This positive pulse is detected when its amplitude is bigger than the selected threshold, which varies between 8/32 and 23/32 of the supply voltage, yielding 16 programmable steps.

Depending on overall system decisions, variations on this structure can be applied, like having a differential input or second comparator to have a window comparator. The circuit applied in the industrial chip design includes a differential input, as shown in Figure 2-7. In this case a buffer is required at the output of the D/A converter that gives the fixed Vbias voltage, since the load is no longer solely the input capacitance of the operational amplifier.

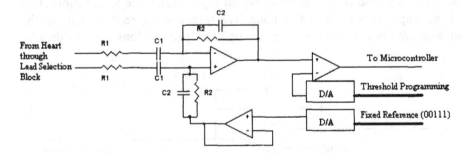

Figure 2-7. Schematic of sense channel in industrial chip with differential input (input clamping diodes not shown)

Let us discuss the characteristics of the selected filter topology. This filter structure allows to implement the desired gain and second order band-pass response based on a single operational amplifier. This is an essential aspect to reduce consumption. Another equally important factor is the reduction of the needed external components. Although, along with classical biquad filter structures with two operational amplifiers, there exist other configurations based on a single amplifier [SED78], they usually require more complex RC networks and to have higher than unity gain becomes more difficult.

The initial drawback with the architecture of Figure 2-6 is that the resulting transfer function when considering an ideal op. amp. can only implement real poles (or equivalently can only implement a quality factor Q lower than ½). The required response corresponds to a transfer function with complex poles and quality factor of 0.9. This issue is solved by letting the frequency response of the amplifier define the low pass characteristic. In this way, complex poles are achieved.

Allowing the amplifier to set the low pass characteristic alone, even C2 can be eliminated. However, in this case the low-pass cut-off frequency is more sensitive to variations of the amplifier's transition frequency (f_T). This conclusion is supported by the results shown later in Table 2-2, where the change in the filter's cut-off frequencies and gain due to changes in f_T for designs with and without C2 are listed. In this table, the filter gain is represented through its effect on the channel sensitivity, i.e. the amplitude of the triangular input signal corresponding to the threshold of detection.

The utility of C2 is twofold. On one hand, the dependence of the frequency response on the amplifier's f_T is reduced. On the other hand, an external way of adjusting the low-pass cut-off frequency is available. This external adjustment is particularly interesting to adjust the frequency response for both the atrial and ventricular channels, while applying the same operational amplifier (hence, the same f_T) in both cases.

1.3.1 External components and amplifier specifications

From the architecture of Figure 2-6, the requirements on its basic components, amplifier and comparator, as well as the values of external components can be derived.

External components and operational amplifier transition frequency (f_T)

These parameters determine the filter response. We will consider in what follows the case of the atrial sensing channel, which is the one handling the smallest signals, hence requiring the highest gain and having the more demanding requirements.

Due to the high closed loop gain, the op amp frequency response influences the low pass filter characteristic at frequencies well below the transition frequency and the non-dominant pole frequency. Therefore, the meaningful parameter to characterize the influence of the op amp frequency response on the overall filter frequency response is the transition frequency of a first order model of the op amp instead of the actual transition frequency, which is influenced by the non-dominant pole. Unless otherwise noted we will refer as f_T to this first order, extrapolated transition frequency. The external components and f_T values applied were: R1 = 22kΩ, C1 = 47nF, R2 = 22MΩ, C2 = 15pF and f_T = 160kHz. This component and f_T selection complies with the following criteria: to provide an input impedance of the filter higher than 20kΩ, as required in the general specifications presented in Chapter 1; to set a high load impedance (high R2 and low C2 values) for the operational amplifier and to approximate the desired frequency response with standard component values. The selected values yield −3dB frequencies of 76Hz and 240Hz and an input threshold voltage step of 0.23mV. The selection of non-standard values for the external component makes it possible to set the frequency limits and threshold voltage step much closer to the initial specification of a 70 to 200Hz frequency band with 0.2mV step. Nevertheless, as analyzed in Chapter 1, this is not critical. The rest of the work applies the standard values presented above.

Table 2-2 quantitatively assesses the benefit of controlling the low pass cut off frequency partly by capacitor C2, instead of letting it be fixed only by the op amp f_T. The filter characteristics considered in Table 2-2 are the −3dB frequencies and the channel sensitivity defined as the necessary amplitude of the triangular test signal in order to reach the detection threshold. Table 2-2 shows, in the first two columns, the effect on these characteristics due to variations of f_T and C2 of respectively ±20% and ±5% around their nominal values (respectively 160kHz and 15pF). Only one parameter is varied in each column and all the other components are fixed at their nominal value. The third column of Table 2-2 addresses the effect of f_T spreads in a design without the C2 capacitor. In this third column, nominal values that yield the same −3dB frequencies and sensitivity as the final design were considered for the rest of the parameters: f_T=120kHz, R1=22kΩ, C1=65nF and R2=16MΩ.

This table shows that the inclusion of C2, besides providing a tuning element for the high cut off frequency, decreases the variation of this frequency with f_T, from around 15% to about 12%.

Load

The load capacitance was specified at 50pF. This value takes into account the parasitic capacitance associated with the off-chip connection and the external C2 feedback capacitance.

The load resistance is given by the feedback resistor R2 (22MΩ) and a 10MΩ resistor to ground to allow for the measurement of the stage operation with an oscilloscope.

Table 2-2. Variation of the filter characteristics (-3dB low and high frequencies and channel sensitivity) due to changes of f_T and C2. All variations are taken around the following nominal values: the first and second columns apply the nominal final design values: f_T=160kHz, C2=15pF, R1=22kΩ, C1=47nF and R2 = 22MΩ; the third column considers nominal values that taking C2 equal to zero, yield the same –3dB frequencies and sensitivity as the final design: f_T=120kHz, R1=22kΩ, C1=65nF and R2=16MΩ.

	Design with C2		Design without C2
	$\Delta f_T = \pm 20\%$	$\Delta C2 = \pm 5\%$	$\Delta f_T = \pm 20\%$
$\Delta f._{3dB}$low (%)	+4.2 / -3.2	+0.87 / -0.86	+4.2 / -5.3
$\Delta f._{3dB}$high (%)	+11 / -12	+0.34/ -0.32	+15 / -15
Δsensitivity (%)	+2.9 / -1.8	+0.75/ -0.75	+3.7 / -2.3

Operational amplifier low frequency gain (A_0)

The low frequency gain (A_0) must be such that the filter response is not too dependent on the A_0 value, which might have a large spread. From the transfer function of the filter of Figure 2-6 it can be observed that the condition to assure that the transfer function is independent of A_0 is that:

$$A_0 \gg \frac{R_2 C_1}{R_2 C_2 + R_1 C_1 + \dfrac{1}{2\pi f_T}} \qquad (2.1)$$

The resulting condition for the above referred values of external components and f_T is $A_0 \gg 757$. The goal for the A_0 gain was set above 10000 (80dB).

Phase margin, slew-rate and load current

When referring to slew-rate it is important to remember that it must be separately considered for each one of the amplifier's stages. Phase margin and load current (which imposes the output stage slew-rate) are dependent on the output stage architecture and current. Hence, we will discuss these three aspects together since requirements on one of these parameters impact on the others.

The required peak output current is given by:

$$I_{load,peak} = V_{out,peak} \left(\frac{1}{R_L} + 2\pi f_{max} C_L \right) \qquad (2.2)$$

where $V_{out,peak}$ is the maximum peak output voltage, R_L and C_L are the resistive and capacitive components of the load and f_{max} is the maximum signal frequency to be delivered at the output without distortion. We will consider $V_{out,peak}$ to be half the supply voltage, which is the span of the detection thresholds at the input of the comparator. The f_{max} frequency will be considered equal to 200Hz, which is the ideal low-pass cut-off frequency of the filter. The resulting maximum load current is 290nA. This definition of f_{max} is more demanding than just considering the case of the triangular test signal. In the case of the triangular test signal, the resulting load peak current is 220nA.

A key issue is that this load current requirement sets a minimum quiescent consumption for the amplifier output stage, unless a class AB output stage is applied, in which case the quiescent current is lower than the maximum output current[1].

The definitions of $V_{out,peak}$ and f_{max} require a slew-rate (SR) of

$$SR = V_{out,peak} \cdot 2.\pi.f_{max} = 1759 \; \frac{V}{s} \qquad (2.3)$$

This slew-rate requirement must be fulfilled by both the amplifier input and output stages. In the case of the output stage, achieving the desired slew-rate is equivalent to complying with the load current requirement previously discussed. In the case of the input stage, the needed slew rate also limits the minimum value of bias current that can be used. However, there is an essential difference with the output stage. If an amplifier with more than one stage is applied -let us consider for instance a two stage Miller amplifier, which will be the one used in our case - the input stage slew-rate will be related to the much smaller Miller capacitor instead of the load capacitor. Consequently, the input stage slew rate requirement is fulfilled with much lower currents than the output stage one. This makes it unnecessary to apply methods to improve the input stage slew rate, such as class AB input stages architectures [CAS852, DEG82].

Regarding the phase margin, an important consumption reduction can be achieved exploiting the fact that the amplifier is intended for application at a fixed feedback condition with high gain. In this configuration, the modulus of the open loop gain of the whole filter will value one when the op amp open loop gain equals the closed loop gain. This happens approximately at the low pass cut off frequency, since this cut off frequency is defined by the

---

[1] This analysis led us to the development of a new approach for the design of a micropower class AB output stage. This micropower class AB output stage is an essential element to achieve extensive current saving in the sense channel implementation presented in Chapter 6.

op amp frequency response. Hence, the phase margin must be evaluated at this frequency. The classical phase margin requirement at the transition frequency, which considers as a worst case a unity gain closed loop gain, is not relevant. Our design criterion was to have the non-dominant pole of the amplifier at least 2 decades after the closed-loop dominant pole frequency (200 Hz), i.e. after 20kHz. This criterion is conservative but has been chosen for two reasons. First, it allows for a safety margin in the load capacitor value. Second, in practice, for all the architectures considered, the load current requirement dominates over this requirement, imposing the non-dominant pole to lie at frequencies slightly higher than 20kHz. Therefore though lower non-dominant poles could be allowed, this fact could not be exploited to further reduce consumption.

Input common mode range

In the architecture of Figure 2-6 the operational amplifier operates at a fixed common mode input voltage of V_{bias}, set at 7/32 of the power supply voltage, i.e. from 0.44V to 0.61V when the power supply ranges from 2V to 2.8V. This input common mode range close to ground suggests the application of a p-type input stage, which is also convenient due to its better 1/f-noise characteristics.

Output swing

The amplifier output must be able to vary from the quiescent point at V_{bias} up to V_{bias} plus half V_{DD}, which is the range of comparison thresholds. Therefore in the worst case condition of 2V power supply, the output swing must be from V_{ss} + 0.44V up to V_{DD} − 0.56. This is not very demanding, as expected, since the selection of the overall architecture took care of easing this aspect.

Common mode rejection ratio

In the case of the architecture of Figure 2-6, there is no common mode signal since the common mode input is fixed at Vbias. This is not the case in a differential topology like the one in Figure 2-7. However in the case of a differential topology the overall filter CMRR requirement is fixed at 40dB and is mainly set by the matching of external components.

Power supply rejection ratio

This specification is not critical since the circuit is powered from a battery and when in operation, no other important source of consumption that might alter the battery voltage is present.

Overall precision: component spread, offset and noise

The overall precision in the threshold of detection depends on several factors. The spread of external components as well as that of the amplifier transition frequency and open loop gain vary the filter gain. The effect of the offset and noise of the op amp and comparator can be modeled as a variation in the level of comparison set by the D/A converter (see Figure 2-6). We will first consider the variation of the filter characteristics due to the expected spread of components and op amp characteristics (f_T and A_0) to then derive the requirements on offset and noise of the op amp and comparator.

Table 2-3 evaluates the variation in the filter characteristics with the spread of external components, amplifier transition frequency and open loop gain.

The filter characteristics considered are the −3dB frequencies and the channel sensitivity defined as the necessary amplitude of the triangular test signal in order to reach the detection threshold. Table 2-3 shows the effect on these characteristics due to variations in R1 of ±1%, in R2 of ±5%, in C1 of ±10%, in C2 of ±5%, in f_T of ±20% and in A_0 of ±10dB around nominal values of, respectively, 22KΩ, 22MΩ, 47nF, 15pF, 160kHz and 85dB. The considered tolerances are, in the case of the external components, those commonly available for the corresponding nominal value (e.g. 22K, 1% resistors are commonly available, but 22MΩ resistors are usually only available at 5% tolerance). For the op amp characteristics, estimated worst case variations based on the spread of process parameters were considered. Only one parameter is varied in each row, all the other components are fixed at their nominal value.

The results of Table 2-3 lead to compound relative variations of the −3dB low and high frequencies that comply with the limits of respectively 10% and 20%, specified in Chapter 1. The variation of the amplifier gain, which is presented in Table 2-3 through the sensitivity variation, is taken into account jointly with the effects of offset and noise, in order to analyze the precision of the detection threshold.

Table 2-3. Variation of the filter characteristics (-3dB low and high frequencies and channel sensitivity) due to changes of R1, R2, C1, C2, f_T and A_0. All variations are taken around the nominal final design values: R1=22kΩ, R2 = 22MΩ, C1=47nF, C2=15pF, f_T=160kHz and A_0 = 85dB.

	Δf_{-3dB}low (%)	Δf_{-3dB}high (%)	Δsensitivity (%)
ΔR1 (± 1 %)	+0.4 / -0.4	+0.19 / -0.19	+0.4 / -0.4
ΔR2 (± 5 %)	+2.0 / -1.9	+3.2 / -3.0	+3.8 / -3.4
ΔC1 (± 10 %)	+7 / -6	+4 / -3	+5 / -4
ΔC2 (± 5 %)	+0.87 / -0.86	+0.34 / -0.32	+0.75 / -0.75
Δf_T (± 20 %)	+4.2 / -3.2	+11 / -12	+2.9 / -1.8
ΔA_0 (± 10 dB)	+1.5 / -4.4	+4.6 / -1.4	+4.6 / -1.4

Offset and noise affect the channel performance as an error in the level of comparison at the input of the comparator. The amplifier offset voltage appears with unity gain at the amplifier output. Hence, it has the same effect as the comparator offset. The amplifiers noise adds up to these two factors, affecting the actual threshold of detection. The comparator's input equivalent noise also adds in the same way, but it will be negligible with respect to the amplifier's output noise and mV level offset voltages.

We will now analyze the relative error in the channel sensitivity S in order to determine the acceptable value of offset and noise. The channel sensitivity S is given by:

$$S = \frac{V_{th}}{G} \tag{2.4}$$

where V_{th} is the nominal selected threshold of detection referred to the quiescent output level of the amplifier (i.e. the difference between the output of the D/A and V_{bias} in Figure 2-6), and G is the gain that relates the amplitude of the input test signal and the output of the filter.

The relative error can be expressed as:

$$\frac{\Delta S}{S} \cong \frac{1}{S}\left(\frac{\partial S}{\partial V_{th}} \Delta V_{th} + \frac{\partial S}{\partial G} \Delta G \right) = \frac{\Delta V_{th}}{V_{th}} - \frac{\Delta G}{G} \tag{2.5}$$

Based on the statistical independence of the threshold variation and the gain variation and assuming a gaussian distribution for both factors, the standard deviation of the relative error in the sensitivity is given by:

$$\sigma\left(\frac{\Delta S}{S} \right) = \sqrt{ \sigma^2\left(\frac{\Delta V_{th}}{V_{th}} \right) + \sigma^2\left(\frac{\Delta G}{G} \right) } \tag{2.6}$$

where $\sigma()$ stands for the standard deviation.

ΔG is related to the variation of sensitivity included in Table 2-3 and ΔV_{th} is determined by offsets and noise. We will now consider how to combine the effects that determine each of these two parameters in order to estimate them.

In the case of ΔG, the worst case for the variations of R1, R2, C1, C2, f_T and A_0 could be considered, but this procedure leads to estimations that are unrealistically pessimistic. Instead we consider that the results included in Table 2-3, which are the maximum, worst case variations due to each parameter, correspond to three times the standard deviation of a gaussian distribution around the nominal value of sensitivity. Then, from the values of Table 2-3 we deduced the standard deviation of the relative variation of gain ($\Delta G/G$) with each parameter. The standard deviation of ($\Delta G/G$) due to the combined effect of all the parameters is determined based on two hypotheses. First, that the parameters are statistically independent, which is assured for the external components and a reasonable hypothesis for f_T and A_0. Second, we assume that for small parameters variations we can approximate the total gain variation as a linear combination of the variation of each parameter, as previously done in the case of the sensitivity as a function of V_{th} and G. Under these assumptions, the standard deviation of ($\Delta G/G$), i.e. $\sigma((\Delta G/G))$ is determined as shown in Eq.(2.7), where δG_i is the relative variation of G due to changes in parameter i.

$$\sigma\left(\frac{\Delta G}{G}\right)=$$

$$\sqrt{\sigma^2\left(\delta G_{R_1}\right)+\sigma^2\left(\delta G_{R_2}\right)+\sigma^2\left(\delta G_{C_1}\right)+\sigma^2\left(\delta G_{C_2}\right)+\sigma^2\left(\delta G_{f_T}\right)+\sigma^2\left(\delta G_{A_0}\right)}$$

$$(2.7)$$

In a similar way, supposing the offsets are purely random (i.e. assuming the systematic offset is negligible, which is usually the case) and taking into account that the three factors (amplifier's offset, comparator's offset and amplifier's noise) will be statistically independent; we can calculate the compound effect of the three factors on $\sigma(\Delta V_{th})$ the standard deviation of the change in the threshold of detection:

$$\sigma(\Delta Vth)=\sqrt{v_{offset,amp}^2 + v_{offset,comp}^2 + v_{nout,amp}^2}\qquad(2.8)$$

where $v_{offset,amp}$ and $v_{offset,comp}$ are respectively the amplifier and comparator offsets, $v_{nout,amp}$ is the rms value of the amplifier's output noise.

If we impose that $\sigma(\Delta V_{th})$ is 20% of the minimum threshold of detection at 2.8V power supply, applying Eq. (2.6) results in a relative error of 20% for the smallest threshold and in an error of less than 10% for the other thresholds. These errors comply with the precision specifications proposed in Chapter 1. If, then, we share this ΔV_{th} error budget in equal parts among the three factors, we have the allowable value for offsets and rms output noise to be 10.1mV. This is a reasonable offset value to aim at, based only on device matching, that does not require the application of any offset cancellation technique.

1.3.2 Amplifier implementation

In the present bulk CMOS IC, the amplifier was implemented as a class A Miller OTA. The internal compensation was a desirable feature in order to have a transition frequency independent from the load capacitor that could have a large spread. This spread is, on the one hand, due to changes in the C2 value, for example when considering the atrial or ventricular channel that require different gain while it is desirable to apply the same internal circuitry. On the other hand, the load capacitance varies due to changes in the parasitic capacitance at the output node. This consideration precludes the application of single stage amplifier architectures like folded cascode, whose transition frequency is fixed by the load capacitance. Furthermore, a cascoded single stage amplifier (a folded cascode or a symmetrical OTA with cascoded output stage) would be very inefficient in terms of power consumption, since, on the one hand, the output stage would require a high bias current (at least 290nA as estimated above) to comply with the load current requirement that was previously discussed. On the other hand, as the transition frequency is set by the high valued load capacitance, the input stage would require a much increased bias current than in the case of the Miller amplifier, where the transition frequency is fixed by the much smaller compensation capacitor.

The total nominal current consumption of the class A Miller OTA is 550nA, 50nA in the bias current input branch, 100nA in the input differential pair and 400nA in the output stage. Input and output stages are biased in moderate inversion to optimize consumption, saturation (V_{DS}) and bias (V_{GS}) voltage and area trade-off. The current mirrors are also biased in moderate inversion in order to increase the output voltage swing while improving matching and offset as discussed in section 3.2 of Chapter 3.

Its main measured characteristics are summarized in Table 2-4.

Table 2-4. Bulk amplifier main characteristics.

Characteristic	Value
A_0	78 dB
Extrapolated first order f_T	160kHz
First Stage Slew Rate	86e3 V/s
Output Stage Slew Rate	8e3 V/s
Consumption	550nA
Die Area	0.21 mm^2

1.3.3   Comparator specifications and implementation

The main comparator specifications are its speed (delay), offset and the input signal range.

Neither the slow varying input signal nor the dynamics of the application, which evolves at "biological" speed, are much demanding on the speed of the comparator. The initial specification for the comparator maximum delay was set at 0.5ms.

The required offset voltage specification was previously estimated to be below 10mV.

The specification regarding the input signal range has strong influence on the selection of the architecture. The architecture of Figure 2-6 requires the comparator to have rail to rail input, or specifically it must be able to handle input signals around half the supply voltage. In the following paragraphs, we will discuss the consequences that this specification has and the novel approach applied for solving it [BAR96].

We can classify comparator topologies according to their principle of operation in three broad classes [ALL84, pp.425 - 437 in GRE86, chapter 4 in VDP94]:

1. based on a high gain amplifier,
2. based on regenerative or positive feedback and
3. other switched-capacitor based architectures.

Let's briefly describe each of these alternatives and evaluate them in light of the above requirements. Topology 1. is typically an open loop op-amp without internal compensation, sometimes in a multistage configuration to increase the speed. The second class of topology takes advantage of the positive feedback of a flip-flop structure to speed up the comparison. Although exceptions exist [ALL84], these circuits usually apply one of the following principles:

1. a switch forces both outputs of the flip-flop to its state of unstable equilibrium and then lets them evolve to the final state according to the difference between the comparator's inputs, or
2. with the flip flop structure turned off, a couple of switches force the outputs to be equal to the comparator inputs (or their amplified version) and then turns on the flip flop that will evolve to the final state.

This structure is discarded because it requires a switch operating in the whole power supply range. The topologies corresponding to the third class as well as the switched-capacitor techniques available to cancel out the comparator offset cannot be applied for the same reason.

Therefore, an op-amp based comparator topology was chosen. The input stage of the op-amp was determined by the rail-to-rail input requirement. The parallel combination of an n and a p differential pair was selected

[HUI85]. The low speed required as well as the high gain achievable operating in weak inversion allow the application of a single-stage structure. Consequently, the amplifier topology shown in Figure 2-8 was considered. It is an adaptation of the well-known "symmetrical OTA" ([KRU81]) structure to the rail-to-rail input stage. The transconductance of this circuit varies with the input common mode voltage level, making the comparator speed to vary accordingly. However, this is not a problem, it just imposes to comply with the required speed for the worst case condition, when only one of the input pairs is operating and the transconductance is at its minimum.

Following the amplifying stage, a minimum sized buffer (to minimize the amplifier load capacitance) is included.

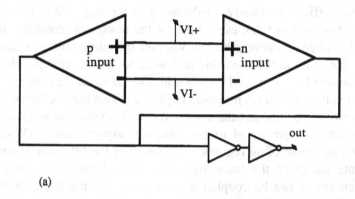

(a)

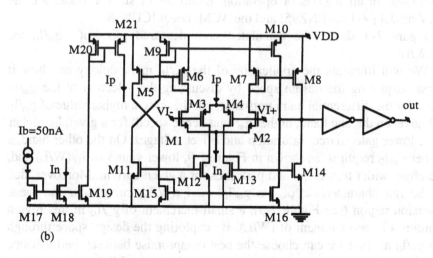

(b)

Figure 2-8. Rail-to-rail comparator (a) basic structure (b) detailed transistor level schematic.

To guarantee the rail-to-rail input operation the following condition must be fulfilled:

$$V_{DD} \geq V_{GSp} - V_{GSn} + 2.V_{DSAT} \qquad (2.9)$$

where V_{DD} is the supply voltage, V_{GSp} and V_{GSn} are the gate source voltage of the p and n input pair transistors and V_{DSAT} is the minimum voltage required across the transistors of the current sources at the source of the differential pairs (M18 and M21) to ensure they are saturated. This condition ensures that the regions of operation of the n and p differential pairs overlap near $V_{DD}/2$ and that a gap where both M18 and M21 are not saturated will not appear.

It may seem difficult to satisfy condition (2.9) for $V_{DD} = 2V$ and the typical threshold voltage of 0.85, even more for the worst case condition of 1.0V threshold voltage. However, the low V_{GS} and saturation voltage values reached when operating in the moderate and weak inversion regions, allow satisfying condition (2.9) even for 1V threshold. The sizing of the transistors was done through the method we proposed in [SIL96]. This method based on the relation between the transconductance over drain current ratio (g_m/I_D) and the drain current normalized to the transistor aspect ratio $I_D/(W/L)$, allows a unified treatment of all regions of operation of the MOS transistors and an accurate sizing of the transistors. The method can be based on experimental curves or can be coupled with an analytical transistor model continuous in all regions of operation. Examples of such a model are the EKV model [VIT93, ENZ95] and the ACM model [CUN98].

Figure 2-9 shows the calculated and measured plots of g_m/I_D vs. $I_D/(W/L)$.

We will illustrate the application of the g_m/I_D methodology and how it allows exploring the design space by discussing the selection of the g_m/I_D value for the differential pairs transistors. In this case a higher value of g_m/I_D will give, on the one hand, higher g_m (and hence speed) for a given I_D, higher gain, lower gate-source, saturation and offset voltages. On the other hand, a higher g_m/I_D requires, as shown in Figure 2-9, lower values of $I_D/(W/L)$ and, therefore, wider transistors and parasitics for a given current. Moreover, due to the flat characteristic of the g_m/I_D vs. $I_D/(W/L)$ curve near the weak inversion region (see Figure 2-9), a small increment of g_m/I_D in this region requires a large increment of (W/L). By exploring the design space through the g_m/I_D method we can choose the best compromise between performance and area. This approach led to a value of $g_m/I_D = 24V^{-1}$ for the input differential pairs transistors, which corresponds to (W/L) of 29 for the nMOS transistors and 69.5 for the pMOS transistors. The resulting V_{GS} value is 0.7V for a threshold voltage V_{T0} of 0.85V and 0.85V for a V_{T0} of 1V. These values of V_{GS} are compatible with condition (2.9) with a 2V power supply and V_{DSAT} corresponding to operation near weak inversion between 0.1 and 0.15V. It is interesting to note that a g_m/I_D value of $25V^{-1}$ (fully in the weak inversion region) leads to (W/L) values of 198 and 477 for the n and p transistor respectively, offering a negligible increase in gain, speed and offset, and V_{GS} at V_{T0} equal to 1.0V is only reduced from 0.85V to 0.77V.

The transistors of current sources and current mirrors are operated in moderate inversion in order to fulfill the low V_{GS} and V_{DSAT} requirement, while improving matching and offset as discussed in section 3.2 of Chapter 3.

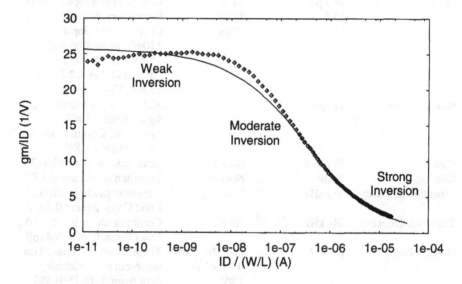

Figure 2-9. Calculated (with the EKV model, solid line) and measured g_m/I_D vs. $I_D/(W/L)$ curve for the applied 2.4μm Bulk CMOS technology.

Experimental and simulation results at 2V power supply are summarized in Table 2-5 and Figure 2-10.

The results of Table 2-5 show that good agreement was reached between expected and measured values for the comparator delay and that a careful layout with a common centroid structure for the differential pairs resulted in a offset value, much lower than the previously estimated requirement of 10mV.

Figure 2-10 shows the evolution of the current consumption with the input common mode voltage. The regions where either one or both differential pairs are operating are clearly visible.

The design meets the challenge posed by the rail-to-rail operation requirement at low supply voltage through a suitable input stage and careful sizing of the transistors for operation in weak and moderate inversion. As will be shown in the following chapters, the characteristics of Fully-Depleted SOI Technology allows us to greatly simplify this structure leading to substantial consumption savings.

Table 2-5. Comparator expected and measured characteristics at 2V supply voltage (unless otherwise noted).

	Design values and simulations results	Measurements	Comments.
Quiescent Current	500 nA maximum	See Figure 2-10	
Delay	24.7 µs	30 µs	Common mode input: 1.915V
	15.5 µs	22 µs	Common mode input: 1.115V
	25.6 µs	30 µs	Common mode input: 0.115V 110mV input step with 15mV overdrive, Ib (shown in Figure 2-8 (b)) = 72 nA, V_{DD} = 2.4V.
Maximum Delay	170 µs		32.5mV input triangular signal with 1.5mV overdrive, Common mode range: 0.2V - 1.8V.
Gain	59 dB	Note 1	Common mode level: 0.3V
Gain	61 dB	Note 1	Common mode level: 1.0V
Transition frequency	235 kHz	Note 1	Common mode level: 0.3V, Load Capacitance: 0.42pF
Transition frequency	344 kHz	Note 1	Common mode level: 1.0V, Load Capacitance: 0.42pF
Offset voltage	6.6 mV	max. 2mV for 0.1V < Vi < 1.9V.	The estimation is based on representative matching data from Refs. [PEL89] and [FOR94]: β standard deviation $\sigma(\Delta\beta/\beta)$=0.2% and V_{T0} standard deviation σ_T=2mV.

Note 1. The output of the amplifying stage is an internal node, not available for measurement externally to the chip (see Figure 2-8).

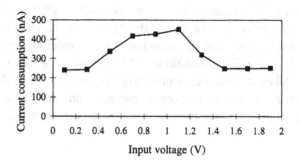

Figure 2-10. Total current consumption vs. input common mode voltage at 2V power supply.

2. CONCLUSIONS

This chapter has presented our implementation of one of the main analog signal processing blocks included in an industrial Bulk CMOS IC for pacemakers: the sense channel.

We have discussed how the architecture selected for the sense channel favors the reduction of power consumption. The selection of architecture is supported on the review of the prior work on implementation of filters with large time constants that is presented in Appendix 1. We derived then the complete specification of the basic modules of the sense channel that will serve as study vehicle for development of new design approaches and implementation in SOI technology in the rest of this work.

In the selected architecture of the sense channel filter/amplifier the OTA transition frequency fixes the cut off frequency of the filter and the OTA must drive a high external load. We have shown that these characteristics make a Miller OTA the most suitable choice. A further improvement to this circuit architecture is presented in Chapter 5, with the introduction of a class AB output stage.

We have shown the challenges for the design of these circuits aiming at operation with 2V power supply in traditional Bulk CMOS technology. These challenges, in our application, are mainly related to the operation of switches and reduced input common mode range of differential stages. We have then illustrated, for the comparator case, how the application of suitable circuit architectures and accurate sizing of the transistors for operation in the weak and moderate inversion regions allow us to solve these challenges. The architectures of these circuits can be simplified based on the superior characteristics of Fully-Depleted SOI technology, reducing power consumption, as will be shown in the following chapters.

Further illustration of the techniques applied to achieve micropower consumption and 2V operation in a standard Bulk CMOS technology are presented in Appendix 2, where the design of the accelerometer signal conditioning circuit is presented, including a new modeling technique for a sample and hold stage. This technique, which is aimed at an oversampling environment, makes it possible to precisely take into account the effect of the switch on-resistance and leakage currents on the stage operation, optimizing the sensor interface to minimize power consumption.

Chapter 3

Potential of SOI Technology for Low-Voltage Micropower Biomedical Applications

Silicon-on-Insulator (SOI) technology has evolved from being exclusively devoted to "niche" market areas as radiation hard or high temperature applications to recently becoming a player in the high performance digital circuits market [IBM011, IBM012]. In addition, the international semiconductor community sees the fully-depleted (FD) variety, which is the one tested in this work, as one of the strong alternatives for solving the transistor scaling challenges in next generations of very deep sub micron processes [ITR01]. We will summarize here the characteristics of the type of SOI MOS devices used in this work, in order to compare later the performance of FD SOI and bulk CMOS analog blocks in low-voltage, micropower applications. This comparison is particularly focused on those blocks and performance aspects that are central to the proposed implementation of our study vehicle, the sense channel, as well as to the implementation of other pacemaker analog blocks. This is the case of the speed and precision of current mirrors, which are essential elements in the class AB stage proposed in Chapter 5, and of OTA characteristics such as the power-bandwidth trade-off, noise and offset.

1. SOI DEVICES

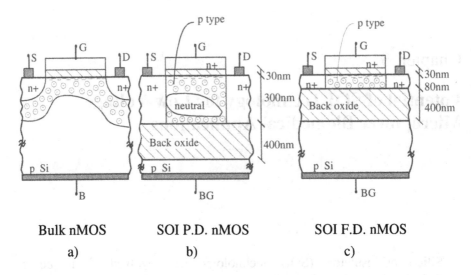

Figure 3-1. Schematic cross sections of Bulk (a), Partially Depleted SOI (b) and Fully Depleted SOI (c) nMOS transistors. Symbols - in a circle denote the depletion region and symbols – represent the inversion layer.

Figure 3-1 a, b and c compares the cross sections of an nMOS transistor in standard, Bulk technology (a) with two main SOI device alternatives, thicker film, partially depleted (PD) and thinner film, fully depleted (FD). In SOI devices, the silicon film, where the transistor action occurs, is built on top of a thick insulator, commonly silicon oxide (named back or buried oxide in opposition to the front thin oxide). This back oxide is in turn on top of a silicon wafer (most commonly, slightly p-type doped) that serves as mechanical support and electrical contact to the back oxide. The contact to the supporting wafer is named back electrode or back gate, since it acts on the device through the back oxide as a secondary gate, common to all the devices of a same die. SOI devices are thus fully, individually isolated by dielectrics, on the contrary to bulk transistors which require isolation by reverse biased junctions and wells.

The best performance of the SOI transistor is obtained with thin film fully depleted devices. In these devices the silicon layer thickness is such that for the practical operating voltages, the front and back depletion layers are merged and the whole silicon layer can be considered depleted, except for the front surface inversion layer that will conduct the transistor current (Figure 3-1 c)). In the case of partially depleted devices, there exists a neutral zone in the silicon layer between the front and back gate depletion regions. Comparing this situation shown in Figure 3-1 b) for the PD SOI transistor and the bulk transistor shown in Figure 3-1 a) we see that the front gate voltage effect on the channel must be much the same. However, the use of PD devices, without a lateral contact to the transistor body to pin the neutral region potential, gives way to detrimental floating body effects such as the so called "kink effect" that degrades the output conductance in saturation of these PD transistors [COL91].

In FD transistors these floating body effects are generally not significant and the absence of a neutral zone results in an improved control of the front gate on the channel [COL91]. This yields a reduced substrate effect which makes the characteristics of FD devices very similar to the characteristics of an ideal MOS transistor. The characteristics of FD transistors show less degradation with temperature than PD and bulk MOS devices.

On the other hand, the thin silicon film applied in FD devices demands for better film quality and uniformity control with respect to what is required in PD devices.

The main advantages of the SOI FD transistor with respect to its Bulk counterpart are [COL91, FLA99]: lower parasitic capacitances, reduced substrate effect, no leakage to substrate, no latch-up in CMOS structures, reduced short channel effects and improved temperature behavior and resistance to radiation-induced transient errors. The drawbacks are lower thermal dissipation capacity leading to self heating effects (which are negligible in low power circuits), lower drain source breakdown voltage and a less mature technology which is less available and more expensive, although this last point is rapidly changing.

We will focus on the first three advantages, which are those that mainly affect the operation and performance of low voltage, micropower analog biomedical circuits that this work deals with. Next, we will proceed to analyze how these differences with standard Bulk technology impact on the characteristics of basic analog modules: switches, current mirrors and operational transconductance amplifiers (OTA).

The increased distance of the active silicon from the substrate through the back oxide reduces the drain and source to substrate capacitances compared to standard bulk technologies. The reduction factor ranges from 3 to 7 in 2μm - 3μm technologies such as those we apply in our experimental prototypes. The reduction factor grows with technology scaling, as long as the back oxide thickness does not need to be scaled, while the bulk parasitic junction capacitances increase with the scaling as the substrate doping is increased to scale the width of the depletion regions. In 0.35μm processes the reduction factor in favor of SOI climbs up to range from 10 to 14. The polysilicon and first metal layer to substrate capacitances are also reduced to a lesser extent (reduction factor from 1.3 to 1.5). A capacitance that is also reduced due to the back oxide layer is the capacitance from the channel to the substrate. This reduction gives way to the improvement in the substrate effect in FD SOI devices. This improvement, which has widespread impact on the characteristics of FD SOI circuits, will be analyzed next.

We will consider the substrate or body effect represented through the parameter that quantifies the coupling between gate voltage and surface potential, thus the effectiveness of the gate voltage to act on the channel. We will refer to this parameter as n, as it is done in analytical models like EKV ([VIT93, ENZ95]) and ACM ([CUN98]) where this parameter plays a central role. The body-effect coefficient or slope factor n is defined as:

$$n = \frac{dV_G}{d\psi_s} \tag{3.1}$$

where V_G is the gate voltage and ψ_s is the surface potential at the front oxide Si-SiO$_2$ interface. Figure 3-2 intuitively depicts the models applied to determine n in a Bulk transistor and a FD SOI transistor ([COL91]). All capacitances shown are per unit area. C_{ox} is the front gate capacitance, C_d is the depletion capacitance, C_{si} is the capacitance of the depleted thin silicon film and C_{oxb} is the SOI back oxide capacitance.

a) Bulk   b) SOI FD

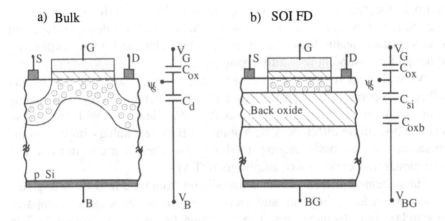

Figure 3-2. Model for determining body-effect coefficient n in Bulk (a) and FD SOI (b).

Applying the model of Figure 3-2 a), the n factor for the bulk transistor case results to be:

$$n = 1 + \frac{C_d}{C_{ox}} \cong 1.4 \text{ to } 1.6 \tag{3.2}$$

in typical 0.7 - 3 μm processes

While for the FD SOI transistor C_d is substituted by the series combination of C_{si} and C_{oxb}, so that:

$$n_{SOI} = 1 + \frac{C_{si}C_{oxb}}{C_{ox} \cdot (C_{si} + C_{oxb})} \underset{(C_{si} \gg C_{oxb})}{\cong} 1 + \frac{C_{oxb}}{C_{ox}} = 1 + \frac{t_{ox}}{t_{oxb}} \approx 1.05 \text{ to } 1.1$$

$$(3.3)$$

where t_{ox} and t_{oxb} are, respectively, the thickness of the front and back oxides. In SOI, as the back oxide capacitance is much smaller than the depletion capacitance of the silicon film, the series of these two capacitances is dominated by the back oxide capacitance. The capacitance "seen" from the channel to the substrate, and consequently the n factor, are much reduced. Besides this reduction, there is a further difference concerning this factor in SOI and Bulk. Since the depletion capacitance C_{si} in SOI is constant while in Bulk it is dependent on the surface potential, in SOI the relationship between gate voltage and surface potential is actually linear while in Bulk the n factor results from a linear approximation of the square root dependence of the depletion capacitance on the surface potential.

The n coefficient defines several important issues for device operation and performance. On the one hand, we have the consequence most widely associated with the body-effect, i.e. the gate-source threshold voltage variation with source to bulk voltage. Besides, this issue, which is mistaken in many traditional presentations of the subject as coinciding with the substrate effect, several other effects on device operation are also associated with the underlying physical phenomenon of the attenuated effect of gate voltage on the channel surface potential, which is referred to as substrate effect. Some of these "macroscopic" effects on device operation, are those appearing on the current drive, the subthreshold slope and the transconductance to current ratio.

The effect of n on the current drive capability of MOS transistors is visible in the following expressions of the drain current of a saturated transistor in the strong inversion (SI) and weak inversion (WI) regions ([ENZ95])

$$\text{SI:} \quad I_D = \frac{\beta}{2n}(V_G - V_{T0} - nV_S)^2 \quad \text{WI:} \quad I_D \propto e^{\frac{(V_G - V_{T0} - n.V_S)}{n.U_T}} \quad (3.4)$$

where β is the product of the mobility μ, C_{ox} and the transistor aspect ratio W/L; V_G and V_S are the gate and source voltages, referred to the substrate in the bulk transistor case and referred to the back gate in the SOI case; V_{T0} is the threshold voltage at zero V_S and U_T is the thermal voltage (kT/q).

It results from the previous expression of the WI drain current in saturation that the inverse subthreshold slope, i.e. $S = \partial V_G / \partial I_D$, is determined by n. Expressed in mV per decade we have:

$$S(mV / dec) = n.U_T \ln(10) \tag{3.5}$$

One joint effect of the increase in subthreshold slope and saturation current is that the threshold voltage can be decreased while preserving the ratio between the transistor on and off currents, as required for correct operation of digital circuits. Figure 3-3 graphically depicts this idea.

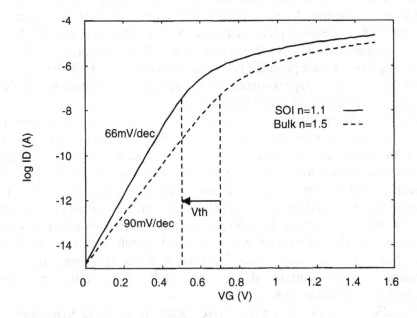

Figure 3-3. Reduction of threshold voltage from 0.7V in Bulk (dashed line) to 0.5V in FD SOI (solid line), while yielding the same off current and increased on current, due to the improved subthreshold slope and current drive capability.

This threshold voltage reduction compatible with digital circuit noise margins leads to FD SOI technologies featuring 0.3V to 0.5V threshold voltages instead of the 0.6 to 0.8V usual in standard Bulk CMOS technologies. This is a factor that, as we will show in several analog circuit blocks and the pacemaker application, makes it possible to either largely reduce minimum required supply voltage or save current, area and design effort thanks to the simplification of the circuit structures required to operate at low supply voltages.

The transconductance to current ratio (g_m/I_D), besides representing the frequency to current efficiency of the device, is intrinsically related to most analog circuit performance aspects. As shown in [SIL96], and further developed below, the following aspects can be determined as function of the g_m/I_D ratio: gain, gate-source and pinch off voltages (and hence amplifiers' input common mode range and output swing), equivalent input thermal noise voltage, offset, current mirror frequency response,....

The maximum value of the g_m/I_D ratio is reached in the WI region and from (3.4), is given by $1/(n.U_T)$. Hence, the decrease in n results in an increase of g_m/I_D in FD SOI, which reaches 35 V^{-1} in WI with respect to 25 V^{-1} for bulk. Figure 3-3 compares the g_m/I_D versus $I_D/(W/L)$ curves for typical 2 μm FD SOI and Bulk technologies. This curve is characteristic of a given process and provides a design tool that relates analog circuit performance (through g_m/I_D) with transistors sizes (through (W/L)) as proposed in [SIL96].

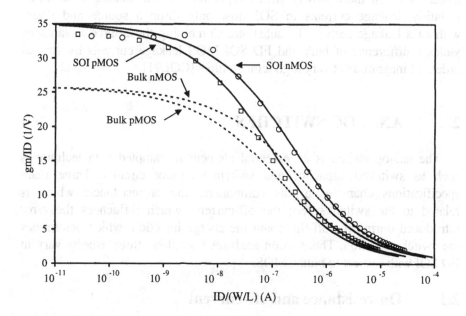

Figure 3-4. Calculated (applying the EKV model [VIT93, ENZ95]) and measured g_m/I_D vs. $I_D/(W/L)$ curves for nMOS and pMOS thin-film SOI fully-depleted transistors and nMOS and pMOS bulk transistors (Calculated SOI: solid line, measured SOI: circles (nMOS), squares (pMOS), calculated bulk: dashed line). From [SIL96], © 1996 IEEE.

The increase in g_m/I_D means an increase in the transconductance generation efficiency of the device, i.e. the ability of translating current (hence power) into transconductance. The transconductance of the device is directly related to the frequency limits of circuits. Therefore, the g_m/I_D value gives us an indication of the speed –power trade-off. This trade-off is further improved in FD SOI due to the reduction of parasitic capacitances. In addition, as the design cases of the following sections will show, these two advantages of FD SOI (lower capacitances and higher g_m/I_D ratio) interplay with the selection of the suitable W/L sizes during the design of complete amplifiers, implying that the overall effect is much higher than just what could be expected from an analysis of the difference between both technologies for a given transistor size.

Since we are interested in circuits that operate with ultra low currents, in the few nA level, a final comment is due regarding leakage current characteristics of FD SOI. Although at room temperature leakage current values in FD SOI and Bulk are comparable, FD SOI presents three significant differences. First, thanks to the reduced film thickness and the absence of wells, SOI devices present much less leaky junction areas. Second, thanks to full depletion operation, the FD SOI leakage current increases much more slowly with temperature. Third, thanks to substrate isolation, leakage currents in SOI flow only through source and drain, without a leakage path to the substrate. Combining these three advantages yields a difference of bulk and FD SOI MOS leakage currents by several orders of magnitude at very high temperatures [COL91].

2.   ANALOG SWITCHES

The analog switch is an essential element in sampled data techniques such as switched capacitor and switched current circuits. Three main specifications characterize this component: the on-resistance, which is related to the switch speed; the off-current, which influences the error introduced during the off-time; and the charge injection, which determines the switch precision. This section analyzes how these three aspects vary in FD SOI with respect to bulk CMOS.

2.1   On-resistance and off-current

In order to handle signals in the whole V_{DD} range, a switch composed by an nMOS and a pMOS transistor connected in parallel is usually applied. The transistor gates are driven by inverted signals as shown in Figure 3-5.

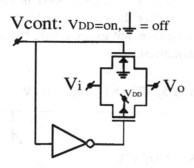

Figure 3-5. Analog CMOS switch. The switch is on when the control signal Vcont is high (voltage equal to V_{DD}), and we apply this voltage on the gate of the nMOS transistor and ground voltage on the gate of the pMOS transistor.

The nMOS transistor on-resistance is lowest for input voltages values V_i near ground, since then the gate-source voltage of the nMOS transistor is maximum. At this point the pMOS transistor does not conduct. As V_i increases, the gate-source voltage of the nMOS transistor decreases, while the source-gate voltage of the pMOS transistor increases. Then the nMOS resistance increases, as it moves towards cut-off, and at some point, the pMOS transistor starts to conduct. As we continue to increase V_i, we finally arrive, near V_{DD}, at a situation that is symmetrical to the initial one: the pMOS transistor fully conducts and the nMOS transistor is cut-off. For V_i values around half V_{DD}, both transistors are supposed to be on. However, as we decrease the supply voltage, we reach a point where the V_i regions where each transistor is on, no longer overlap.

This situation is depicted in Figure 3-6

The minimum supply voltage to guarantee that this conduction gap does not occur depends on the threshold voltage and the n parameter, due to its influence on the dependence of the threshold voltage on the source-to-substrate voltage. This minimum voltage is given by [VIT93]:

$$V_{DD\,min} = \frac{n_n |V_{T0p}| + n_p V_{T0n}}{n_n + n_p - n_n n_p} = \frac{2V_{T0}}{2 - n} \text{ if } |V_{T0p}| = V_{T0n}, n_n = n_p \quad (3.6)$$

The reduced substrate effect of FD SOI, contributes to improve the V_{DDmin} in two ways. First, the threshold voltage increases less with V_i, which is reflected in Eq. (3.6) through a lower n value. Second, lower V_{T0} values can be applied while keeping acceptable levels of off-current. We will analyze these two effects in the following paragraphs.

The actual minimum supply voltage needed is higher than the value provided by Eq. (3.6), since for the circuit to operate correctly, it must be assured not only that there does not exists a gap, but also that a minimum conductance value is guaranteed.

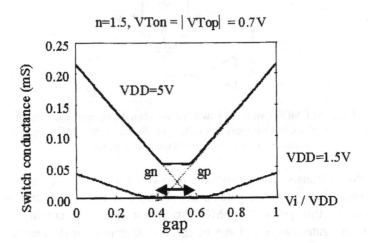

Figure 3-6. Bulk CMOS switch on conductance as a function of input voltage and supply voltage (n=1.5, $V_{T0n} = V_{T0p}$=0.7V). The conductance of the nMOSFET (gn) and pMOSFET (gp) are shown together with their sum, which is the total switch conductance. A gap in conduction is shown for V_{DD} equal to 1.5V.

Figure 3-7 shows the V_{DD} dependence of the maximum symmetrical threshold voltage (V_{T0}=V_{T0n}= V_{T0p}) required to feature a maximum value of on resistance equal to 50kΩ for $0 \leq V_i \leq V_{DD}$. A 50kΩ on resistance is a typical value corresponding to a maximum settling error of 0.01% for a 500kHz clock frequency and a 2pF capacitance. The switch considered has $(W/L)_n$=1 and $(W/L)_p$= 2.5 $\approx (\mu_n/\mu_p)$. This selection of relative sizes for the n and p transistors will be later shown as the one that optimizes the trade-off between signal dependent charge injection error and on-resistance. The computation was performed using the EKV [VIT93, ENZ95] model with n=1.1 in the SOI case and n=1.5 in the bulk case and μ_nC_{ox}=50μA/V^2 and μ_pC_{ox}=20μA/V^2 in both cases.

We observe that the required bulk threshold voltage should become extremely low for reduced V_{DD} in order to maintain sufficient conductance in the mid V_i range. The corresponding bulk off-current then exceeds the maximum admissible current which limits to 0.01% the relative error due to the discharge of the capacitance during the holding phase, as shown in Figure 3-8, which still considers a 500kHz clock frequency with a duty cycle of 0.5.

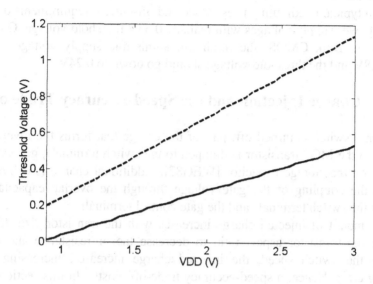

Figure 3-7. Symmetrical threshold voltage for a maximum on-resistance of 50kΩ in SOI (dashed line) and Bulk (solid line). The aspect ratio of the n and p transistors of the switch are respectively $(W/L)_n=1$ and $(W/L)_p = 2.5$ (approximately equal to the ratio of the electrons mobility to the holes mobility).

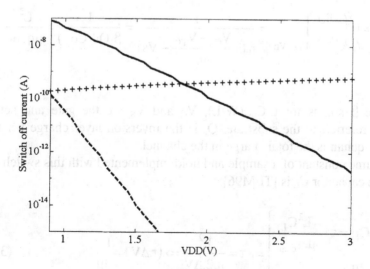

Figure 3-8. Bulk (solid line) and SOI (dashed line) switch off-currents resulting from the threshold voltages of Figure 3-7 as a function of the supply voltage. Also represented is the limit corresponding to a 0.01% error due to the discharge of a 2pF capacitance during a 1μs holding phase (+symbols).

These results show that FD SOI can assure switch operation compatible with both typical maximum on-resistance and off-current requirements down to 1.2V power supply voltages with realistic 0.33V threshold voltage. On the contrary, in Bulk CMOS, the minimum admissible supply voltage stays above 1.8V and the threshold voltage should go down to 0.24V.

2.2   Charge Injection and the Speed-Accuracy Trade off

When a switch is turned off, part of the charge that forms the inversion channel in the MOS transistor is dumped to the switch terminals, generating an error on the storage capacitor [WEG87]. Additional charge is delivered through the coupling of the gate voltage through the overlap capacitance between the switch terminals and the gate control terminal.

The amount of injected charge increases with the transistor size. If we increase the transistor aspect ratio to decrease the on-resistance and thus increase the switch speed, the injected charge increases, increasing the resulting error. Hence, a speed-accuracy trade-off exists. In this section we will analyze this trade-off and compare the cases of SOI and Bulk technologies.

The on-resistance of an MOS transistor operating as a switch, and considering strong inversion operation,   is given by ([VIT93, ENZ95, TEM96]).

$$R_{on} = 1 / \left(\frac{\partial I_D}{\partial V_S} \right)_{V_S \cong V_D} = \frac{1}{n.\beta(\frac{V_G - V_{T0}}{n} - V_S)} = \frac{1}{\beta(Q_i'/C_{ox})} = \frac{L^2}{\mu q_{chan}}$$

$$(3.7)$$

where β stands for $\mu.C_{ox}.(W/L)$, V_G and V_S are the gate and source voltages referred to the substrate, Q_i' is the inversion layer charge per unit area and q_{chan} is the total charge in the channel.

The time constant of a sample and hold implemented with this switch and a storage capacitor C_L is [TEM96]:

$$\left. \begin{array}{c} R_{on}C_L = \tau = \frac{L^2 C_L}{\mu.q_{chan}} \\ \\ \Delta V = \frac{q_{chan}}{2.C_L} \end{array} \right\} \Rightarrow \tau = \frac{L^2}{\mu.2.\Delta V} \Rightarrow (\tau.\Delta V) = \frac{L^2}{2\mu} \qquad (3.8)$$

where ΔV is the error due to charge injection, neglecting the overlap capacitances and assuming the charge is equally distributed to both sides of the switch (which is the case when the turn off of the switch is fast enough [WEG87]).

Eq. (3.8) shows that the speed-accuracy trade-off depends, in first approximation, only on the mobility (a physical constant if we neglect second order effects) and the minimum channel length of the process. Hence, there will not exist from this point of view much difference between Bulk and SOI. However, a different panorama arises if we consider the *signal dependent* part of the charge injection error. This is of interest because we can get rid of the constant component of the error at the system level or by using circuit techniques such as fully differential structures.

Now we will consider the signal dependent part of the charge injection error for the complementary switch, shown in Figure 3-5.

The complete expression of the charge injection error (neglecting weak inversion conduction) for a single transistor switch is given by [WEG87]:

$$\Delta V_{tot} = \text{kov} \frac{2C_{ov}}{C_L}(V_H - V_L) + \text{kchan}\left[\frac{q_{chan}}{C_L}\right] =$$

$$= \text{kov} \frac{2C_{ov}}{C_L}(V_H - V_L) + \text{kchan}\left[\frac{\text{CoxWL}(V_H - V_{T0} - nV_i)}{C_L}\right] \qquad (3.9)$$

where C_{ov} is the gate - source and gate - drain overlap capacitance, kov and kchan are the charge distribution coefficients of the overlap and channel charge to both sides of the switch, V_H and V_L are the on and off values of the gate voltage, and V_i is the voltage that is switched.

When the switch of Figure 3-5 is considered we have the following properties:

a) The offset (constant) parts of the error due to the n and p transistors have opposite sign and hence tend to cancel out.

b) The signal dependent parts of the error due to the n and p transistors *add*.

The resulting maximum signal dependent error is given by:

$$\Delta V_{s.d.max} = \frac{k_{chan}}{C_L} \frac{V_{imax}}{2}\left(n_p W_p L_p C_{oxp} + n_n W_n L_n C_{oxn}\right) \qquad (3.10)$$

where V_{imax} is the maximum value of V_i, the minimum value of V_i is supposed equal to 0 and the 1/2 factor comes from considering variations around the mean value $(V_{imax} - V_{imin})/2 = V_{imax}/2$.

By analyzing the expression of the on-resistance of the parallel combination of the nMOS and pMOS transistors (based on Eq.(3.7)) and Eq. (3.10) for the charge injection error, we have demonstrated that the combination of p and n sizes that gives the minimum signal dependent error with minimum value of the maximum Ron of the switch is:

$$\frac{(W/L)_p}{(W/L)_n} = \frac{n_n \cdot \mu_n}{n_p \cdot \mu_p} \tag{3.11}$$

The rigorous proof will not be included here since it is tedious and does not add much to the understanding of the subject. Instead, we will describe the essential idea behind this result as follows. Letting aside the factor (n_n/n_p) that comes from the expression of the error of Eq. (3.10), the above condition assures that both transistors equally contribute to the maximum resistance of the switch. If that were not the case, the maximum resistance would be fixed by the transistor with smallest current capacity (smallest $\mu.(W/L)$ factor), while the charge injection error is determined by the contribution of both transistors and particularly by the contribution of the one with the biggest (W/L) factor. Therefore, the optimum solution is that given by Eq. (3.11).

With the p and n transistors sized according to Eq. (3.11) and if $n_n = n_p$ and $V_{Ton} = V_{Top}$, the maximum time constant times the signal dependent error is given by:

$$\tau_{max} \Delta V_{s.d.max} = \frac{L^2 k_{chan}}{2} \left(\frac{1}{\mu n} + \frac{1}{\mu p} \right) \frac{V_{DD} \cdot n}{2 \left(V_{DD} \left(1 - \frac{n}{2} \right) - V_{T0} \right)} \tag{3.12}$$

The above formula was derived considering the maximum value of τ (corresponding to the value of V_i that gives maximum on resistance, which, supposing equal n and V_{T0} values for p and n, corresponds to $V_{DD}/2$) and the maximum value of the signal dependent error, which from Eq. (3.10) corresponds to the maximum V_i amplitude (taken equal to V_{DD}).

In order to evaluate the gain that SOI technology can provide to the speed – accuracy trade-off of analog switches, the ratio of the bulk to SOI figures of merit of Eq. (3.12) was evaluated as function of V_{DD}, and respective Bulk and SOI V_{T0} and n values. The threshold voltage for each technology was taken so that the off current is equal to the acceptable limit applied in Figure 3-8. The result is shown in Figure 3-9. This is a result for technologies with hypothetical V_{T0} values. To consider a comparison based on existing processes, some typical cases, which also comply with the off current limit applied in Figure 3-8, are compared in Table 3-1.

These results demonstrate that in SOI technology the supply voltage range of operation of analog switches is widely extended. In addition, even at supply voltages that assure correct operation of Bulk switches, the lower n factor and threshold voltage compatible with acceptable levels of off-current of FD SOI result in a highly relaxed speed accuracy trade-off, which makes it possible to operate at higher speed, precision levels or both.

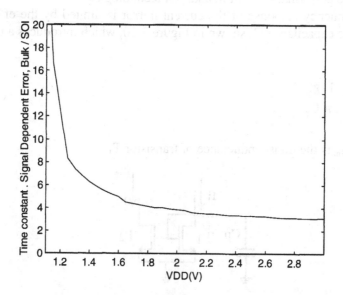

Figure 3-9. Ratio (Bulk over FD SOI) of speed – accuracy trade-off figures of merit of analog switches (i.e. time constant multiplied by the signal dependent charge injection error as given by Eq. (3.12)). The minimum threshold voltages that assures, in each technology, that the off-current is below the limit applied in Figure 3-8 are considered.

Table 3-1. Comparison of speed – accuracy trade-off in Bulk and SOI for typical supply and threshold voltage values.

V_{DD} (V)	V_{T0} Bulk (V)	V_{T0} SOI (V)	$(\tau \Delta V_{s.d.})$max Bulk / $(\tau \Delta V_{s.d.})$max SOI
3	0.7	0.4	26
3	0.6	0.3	9.5
2.5	0.5	0.3	9.0

3.   CURRENT MIRRORS

We will now consider the frequency response and precision of a current mirror.

3.1   Frequency response

First, an expression that relates the current mirror pole frequency with the selected g_m/I_D ratio or transistor inversion level will be developed. This expression is a useful design tool. In addition, it will also allow us to compare the performance in Bulk and SOI technologies.

The frequency response of the current mirror is limited by the effect of the parasitic capacitance C_p shown in Figure 3-10, which introduces a pole at frequency:

$$f_{pole} = \frac{1}{2\pi} \frac{g_m}{C_p}$$ (3.13)

where g_m is the transconductance of transistor T_1.

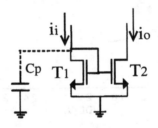

Figure 3-10. Current mirror showing parasitic capacitance Cp that determines the current mirror pole.

Neglecting additional parasitic capacitances due to other circuits connected to the input of the mirror, C_p is equal to:

$$C_p = C_{gs1} - C_{gb1} - C_{gs2} - C_{gb2} - C_{db1} = C_g - C_{db1}$$ (3.14)

i.e. the sum of the total gate to source and substrate capacitances of transistors 1 and 2 (which we will refer to as C_g) and the drain to substrate, extrinsic capacitance of T_1. In the case of SOI the substrate refers to the back gate which is a fixed voltage with respect to ground.

The drain to substrate capacitance has the usual expression:

$$C_{db1} = C_j.W.X - C_{jsw}(2W - 2X) \tag{3.15}$$

where W is the width of T_1, X the extension of the drain contact area of T_1, C_j is the drain –substrate bottom capacitance per unit area and C_{jsw} is the drain – substrate sidewall capacitance per unit perimeter length.

The gate capacitance C_g is proportional to the transistors' gate areas W.L and is a function of the inversion level of the transistors. Considering the mirror has a current gain factor b (i.e. that $W_2 = b. W_1$), C_g can be expressed as:

$$C_g = (1 - b).f(i_f).W.L \tag{3.16}$$

where $f(i_f)$ is a function that describes the dependence of C_g with the inversion level in forward saturation i_f for the transistor. The function $f(i_f)$ is available from analytical models of the MOS transistor that provide a continuous representation in all regions of inversion, such as the EKV model ([VIT93, ENZ95]) and the ACM model ([CUN98]). The inversion level i_f is proportional to the normalized current $I_D/(W/L)$ applied in the g_m/I_D method ([SIL96]), and is defined as follows for the EKV and the ACM model:

$$i_{fEKV} = \frac{I_D}{2n\mu C_{ox}\frac{W}{L}U_T^2} = \frac{i_{fACM}}{4} \tag{3.17}$$

Values of i_f much greater than one indicate operation in strong inversion; those much smaller than one are associated to operation in the weak inversion region and the moderate inversion region falls around i_f equal to one.

Combining equations (3.13) to (3.17), and taking into account that the transconductance g_m is equal to g_m/I_D multiplied by I_D, the current mirror pole can be expressed as:

$$w_{pole} = \frac{\left(g_m/I_D\right)I_D}{(1+b)f(i_f)WL + C_j.W.X + C_{jw}.2.W + C_{jw}2X}$$

$$\cong \frac{\left(g_m/I_D\right)\frac{I_D}{(W/L)}}{(1+b)f(i_f)L^2 + C_j.L.X + C_{jw}.2.L} = g\left(b, \frac{g_m}{I_D}, technology\right) \tag{3.18}$$

The second approximate equality of Eq. (3.18) was obtained neglecting the part of the sidewall drain – substrate capacitance that corresponds to the term $C_{jw}.2X$ and taking as common factor for the denominator the term (W/L).

This expression of the current mirror pole is new, as far as we know, and has some interesting features. It depends only on the g_m/I_D ratio chosen for the transistor (or equivalently the inversion level i_f), the chosen transistor length and parameters related to the technology. Therefore it can be applied to determine the maximum allowable g_m/I_D ratio (or minimum inversion level) for a given frequency requirement. We are assuming here that the length is taken to the minimum to favor frequency response. If this were not the case, Eq. (3.18) will nevertheless allow us to take into account the effect of a non-minimum length selection.

Caution must be taken when applying Eq. (3.18). It does not consider the additional parasitic capacitance that other circuits might add at the mirror input and it would not be accurate in deep strong inversion where velocity saturation affects the transconductance value. Nevertheless, it must be noted that the additional parasitic capacitances that would add to what is considered in Eq. (3.18) are mainly drain –substrate extrinsic capacitances. These capacitances are lower in SOI with respect to Bulk in a bigger proportion than what the total C_p capacitance considered in Eq. (3.18) is. This is so because C_p has one term related to the gate oxide thickness, which would not change from Bulk to SOI. Therefore, the error in the Bulk vs. SOI comparison that results from neglecting these capacitances is attenuated.

Figure 3-11 and Figure 3-12 show the results of applying the expression of Eq. (3.18) to an nMOS current mirror with unity gain (b=1) for the 3µm FD SOI technology of the Université catholique de Louvain (UCL), Belgium ([FLA01]) and a comparable Bulk technology. The data of the technologies are the following: in the UCL SOI technology (resp. Bulk) n=1.1 (1.5), C_{jn} = 0.06 fF/µm^2 (0.18 fF/µm^2), C_{jp} = 0.06 fF/µm^2 (0.4 fF/µm^2), C_{jswn} = 0.05 fF/µm (0.4 fF/µm), C_{jswp} = 0.05 fF/µm (0.5 fF/µm). All other technology data are supposed to be the same for both technologies: the gate oxide thickness (t_{ox} = 30nm), the effective mobility (μ_n=500.10^{-4} m^2/(V.s), μ_p=190e-4 m2/(V.s)), the drain and source region extensions (X_n=X_p=8µm), the source - gate and drain - gate overlap (ov_n = ov_p= 0.15 µm) and the Early voltages (V_{An}= V_{Ap}= 20 V @ 3 µm length).

These results show that an increase in the pole frequency from about 3 times in WI to about 2 times in SI is achieved in FD SOI. If we consider a fixed g_m/I_D ratio of 5 (representative of a "high frequency" oriented design in strong inversion), the resulting pole frequencies are 195 MHz for SOI and 90 MHz for Bulk, an increase by a factor 2.1. This does not even consider the effect of the threshold voltage and voltage swings differences in Bulk and

SOI. On the one hand the lower threshold voltage of FD SOI technology makes it possible to operate the mirror in stronger inversion than in Bulk, while preserving the output swing and input voltage ranges. This would provide important additional frequency gains. On the other hand, we can have the same pole frequency in SOI as in Bulk while operating in weaker inversion. This added to the lower threshold voltage leads to much increased voltage ranges in SOI, for the same frequency characteristics.

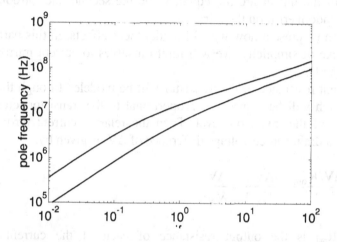

Figure 3-11. Current mirror pole frequency as a function of the transistors' inversion level if for 3μm Bulk (solid line) and FD SOI (dashed line) technologies.

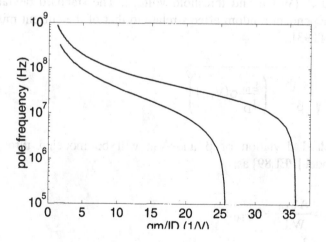

Figure 3-12. Current mirror pole frequency as a function of the transistors' g_m/I_D ratio for 3μm Bulk (solid line) and FD SOI (dashed line) technologies.

The expression of Eq. (3.18) will be applied as design tool in Chapters 4 and 5.

3.2   Precision

Next we consider the precision of the current mirror. Two effects are taken into account; the transistor finite output resistance and mismatch. The first effect introduces an error when the drain source voltages of both transistors of the mirror are not equal, while the second one introduces an additional random error on the mirror gain.

We will now present how we will model these effects. In this part of the study for sake of simplicity, we will limit ourselves to current mirrors with unity gain (b=1).

The output resistance of the transistor will be modeled through the Early voltage, which will be considered proportional to the transistor length and independent of the inversion level. Then the relative current error in the mirror with a drain source voltage difference of ΔV, is given by:

$$\frac{\Delta I}{I} = \frac{\Delta V / R_{out}}{I} = \frac{\Delta V}{V_A} \frac{I}{I} = \frac{\Delta V}{V_A} \qquad (3.19)$$

where R_{out} is the output resistance of each of the current mirror transistors, which is modeled as the Early voltage V_A over the drain current I.

The mismatch of the transistors will be characterized by the mismatch in β (equal to $\mu.C_{ox}(W/L)$) and threshold voltage. The standard deviation of these two independent random effects relate to that of the current mismatch as follows [VIT93]:

$$\sigma\left(\frac{\Delta I}{I}\right) = \sqrt{\frac{\sigma^2(\beta)}{\beta^2} + \left(\frac{g_m}{I_D}\sigma(V_{T0})\right)^2} \qquad (3.20)$$

The standard deviation of β and V_{T0} will be modeled through the Pelgrom's model [PEL89] as:

$$\sigma^2(V_{T0}) = \frac{A_{VT0}^2}{W.L} + S_{VT0}^2.D^2$$

$$\frac{\sigma^2(\beta)}{\beta^2} = \frac{A_\beta^2}{W.L} + S_\beta^2.D^2 \qquad (3.21)$$

where D is the distance between the transistors and A_β, A_{VT0}, S_{VT0} and S_β are coefficients that characterize the matching properties of the particular process. Table 3-2 shows the value of these coefficients for a 2.5μm n-well Bulk technology as reported in [PEL89]. Since these data correspond to a process with similar feature size as the ones we are comparing, these values will be considered in our analysis for both Bulk and SOI technologies. Previous works support the fact that SOI technology matching is comparable to that of classical bulk technologies. Values of $A_{VT0} = 13\text{mV}.\mu\text{m}$ and $A_\beta = 5\%.\mu\text{m}$ have been reported for a 2 μm SOI industrial process ([POR98, EGG98]).

Table 3-2. Matching parameters for 2.5μm Bulk technology taken from [PEL89]

Parameter	nMOS	pMOS
A_{VT0} (mV . μm)	30	35
S_{VT0} (μV / μm)	4	4
A_β (%. μm)	2.3	3.2
S_β (10^{-6} / μm)	2	2

The distance D is very dependent on the layout style and transistor size. On the other hand, as can be seen from the data in Table 3-2, the second terms, (which are those related to the distance) in the right side of Eqs. (3.21) are negligible with respect to the first term for usual small sized mirror transistors. Nevertheless, in the following analysis we considered a first approximation to take into account the effect of the transistor size on the distance between the mirror transistors. This approximation is to assume the transistor layout was such that it gave an approximately square structure for each transistor, with an area approximated by W.L, and so we estimated D as the square root of W.L.

Based on these models, the evolution of the current mirror precision was evaluated in Bulk and SOI as follows. The objective was to evaluate the trade off between precision and consumption for a given target frequency that was chosen at 10MHz. The drain voltage difference between the mirror transistors (ΔV in Eq. (3.19)) was taken equal to 0.5V. Three transistor lengths were considered (3, 6 and 9 μm). For each of these lengths, the g_m/I_D ratio that gave the target 10MHz pole frequency, was determined as discussed in the previous section. Once the g_m/I_D ratio is fixed an additional degree of freedom remains: either the current or the transistor width. We selected to vary the transistor width between 3μm and 30μm and we calculated the resulting current and total error. The total error was defined as the sum of the error due to the output resistance given by Eq. (3.19) plus the standard deviation of the error due to matching, given by Eq. (3.20).

The results are summarized in Table 3-3 and Figure 3-13. Figure 3-13 plots for each of the transistor lengths the current mirror error as a function of the current. The component of the error due to the output resistance, which depends only on the transistor length and decreases with increasing length, is represented by the three horizontal lines plotted in Figure 3-13.

In Table 3-3 we analyze the current savings that are achieved in SOI for a given error target for each of the selected transistor lengths.

Table 3-3. g_m/I_D ratios and drain current required for SOI and Bulk current mirrors with 10MHz pole frequency and the given values of transistor length and total error,. The error considers the matching error and the error due to the output resistance with a 0.5V voltage difference between the drains of the current mirror transistors.

L (μm)	Error (%)	g_m/I_D Bulk (1/V)	g_m/I_D SOI (1/V)	I_D Bulk (nA)	I_D SOI (nA)	I_DBulk / I_DSOI
3	5	19	33	175	50	3.5
6	3	11	20	362	203	1.8
9	2	6	11	860	602	1.4

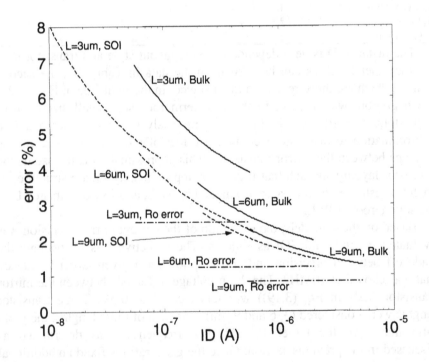

Figure 3-13. Total error of current mirror as a function of drain current for the transistors lengths shown, with 10MHz pole frequency, in SOI (dashed lines) and Bulk (solid lines). The total error considered includes the matching error and the output resistance error for a difference of 0.5V between the current mirror transistor drains. The horizontal, dash-dot lines shown are the error due to the output resistance, which depends only on the transistor length and decreases for increasing length.

These results can be interpreted as follows. As shown in Figure 3-11, for a given pole frequency the SOI mirror can operate closer to weak inversion, i.e. with a smaller inversion coefficient. Hence, for a given transistor size (and thus a given error) the resulting current decreases.

The application of the Pelgrom's matching model jointly with the g_m/I_D methodology, besides making possible a thorough comparison between SOI and Bulk technologies as previously shown, leads to the following interesting result concerning the design of current mirrors.

The transistor W.L product, which defines the standard deviation of β and V_{T0} according to (3.21), can be written as follows, by simultaneously dividing and multiplying by L, I_D and g_m, and rearranging the terms.

$$WL = \frac{W}{L} \cdot \frac{1}{I_D} \cdot I_D \cdot \frac{1}{g_m} \cdot g_m \cdot L^2 = \frac{g_m \cdot L^2}{\left(\dfrac{g_m}{I_D}\right)\left(\dfrac{I_D}{\dfrac{W}{L}}\right)} \tag{3.22}$$

Applying this expression in equations (3.21) and neglecting the terms related to the distance D between the transistors, the standard deviation of the current mismatch, of Eq. (3.20) is given by:

$$\sigma\left(\frac{\Delta I}{I}\right) = \sqrt{\frac{A_\beta^2 + \left(\dfrac{g_m}{I_D}\right)^2 A_{V_{T0}}^2}{g_m L^2}} \left(\frac{g_m}{I_D}\right)\left(\frac{I_D}{\dfrac{W}{L}}\right) =$$

$$= \sqrt{\frac{A_\beta^2 \dfrac{I_D}{\dfrac{W}{L}} + \left(\dfrac{g_m}{I_D}\right)^2 \dfrac{I_D}{\dfrac{W}{L}} A_{V_{T0}}^2}{I_D L^2}} \tag{3.23}$$

The factors ($I_D/(W/L)$) and ($(g_m/I_D)^2 \cdot I_D/(W/L)$) are maximum in strong inversion and minimum in weak inversion. This is so, because as we move from weak to strong inversion, the exponential increase of the normalized current by 3 to 5 orders of magnitude induces a decrease in g_m/I_D by only one order of magnitude (see Figure 3-4). Therefore, if the current and transistor length are fixed, the minimum current mismatch is achieved in weak inversion. This happens because, as the operating point is moved towards weak inversion for a given current, the transistor size increases, leading to a reduction in the spread of β and V_{TO}. This improvement in the matching of bigger transistors dominates over the increase in g_m/I_D occurring due to operation in weaker inversion, which, as predicted by Eq. (3.20), tends to increase the current error. An analysis, only based on Eq. (3.20), leads to the, usual, contrary conclusion: that the best current mirror matching is achieved in strong inversion. This is true when we are considering a *given transistor size*, and hence, given matching characteristics, and we analyze the effect of changing the current. On the contrary, from a design perspective, if the current is fixed and the size is to be determined, Eq. (3.23) shows the best results are achieved when the transistors are designed for operation close to weak inversion. This is, for example, usually the case when the current mirror that loads a differential pair is to be designed; the current is fixed by the design of the differential pair and the length of the current mirror transistors is chosen based on the required bandwidth or gain. The benefit achieved by moving towards deep weak inversion is limited by the fact that in Eq. (3.23) we are neglecting the second terms related to the distance between the matched transistors. These distance related terms tend to increase the mismatch as the transistors get bigger. However, they only are meaningful for very big transistors. Considering the data of Table 3-2, and approximating the distance D by the square root of W.L; a W.L value of 2300 μm^2 is required so that the greatest of these distance related terms equals one tenth of the first, area related, terms of Eqs. (3.21). Considering a 3 μm length, this means a W over L ratio of 767.

Additional limits for the operation in weak inversion are the reduction of the mirror bandwidth (as discussed in the previous section) and the increase of die area.

An exception to the previous analysis occurs when the operation point is moved towards strong inversion by increasing the transistor length. In this case, similar matching as in weak inversion can be achieved for a given current and pole frequency. The price, which in the weak inversion region is paid in the area occupied, here is paid in a decrease in the signal ranges due to increased gate-source and saturation voltages.

4.   OPERATIONAL TRANSCONDUCTANCE AMPLIFIERS

We will now consider the impact of FD SOI technology on the performance of OTAs, particularly those intended for low supply voltage and micropower consumption.

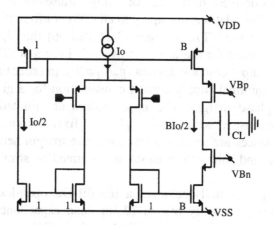

Figure 3-14. Cascoded symmetrical SOI OTA considered for comparison of Bulk and SOI technologies.

This study of the performance of OTAs in FD SOI technology has been pioneered by the UCL SOI group ([FLA94, FLA96]). In this section we will describe our experience [SIL96, section 4 in ref. FLA99] with the cascoded symmetrical OTA of Figure 3-14.

4.1   DC Gain and Transition Frequency

The main results come from the relationship of the g_m/I_D ratio with many central performance parameters of OTAs (gain, transition frequency, output swing, noise ....). This can be appreciated from the following expressions of the gain and transition frequency of a simple common source amplifier loaded by a capacitor C_L and biased with a current source I_D:

$$A_0 = -\frac{g_m}{I_D} V_A \qquad f_T = \frac{1}{2\pi} \frac{g_m}{C_L} \qquad (3.24)$$

where g_m is the small signal transconductance and V_A is the Early voltage that fixes the small signal drain conductance $g_d = I_D/V_A$. Hence, the g_m/I_D

ratio determines the gain and the relation between transition frequency (which is proportional to g_m) and consumption (given by I_D). In addition to the gain improvement derived from the increased g_m/I_D ratio of FD SOI technology (shown in Figure 3-4), the smaller parasitic capacitances of SOI, make it possible to achieve a given phase margin with bigger transistors (higher W/L). This increase in (W/L) translates in an additional increment of g_m/I_D for a given current or f_T.

Eq. (3.24) was derived for the case of a single transistor, common source amplifier, but similar relationships apply to all OTA configurations.

In the design of the OTA of Figure 3-14 [SIL96] the highest possible g_m/I_D values were used for the active transistors, i.e. input differential pair ($g_m/I_D = 28$) and output cascode devices ($g_m/I_D = 30$), in order to optimize the performance for minimal supply current consumption for a given transition frequency and phase margin. The upper values are limited by stability considerations because as we increase g_m/I_D for a fixed current, the transistor sizes and capacitances are increased and the phase margin hence decreased. The bias current and mirror transistors are operated in stronger inversion ($g_m/I_D = 8$).

This OTA experimentally achieved a 103 dB DC open-loop gain and a 271 kHz transition frequency over a 12.3pF load capacitance with a 60° phase margin and a total current of 2µA under a 3V power supply, in accordance with the targeted and simulated specifications. The output swing was almost equal to 2V. We estimated that to achieve a similar f_T performance with same C_L and phase margin, the bulk implementation could have only used g_m/I_D ratios of 19 and 17 for the input differential pair and output cascode transistors respectively and would have dissipated 45% more supply current for a DC open loop gain reduced by 8dB.

In addition, we took advantage of the easy exploration of the design space provided by the g_m/I_D method, in order to analyze the evolution of the bulk and SOI implementations of the OTA as a function of the specified transition frequency for the same phase margin of 60°. As higher transition frequencies were sought, all the transistors were taken of minimum length (3 µm) in both SOI and bulk implementations, and the g_m/I_D of the current mirrors was taken equal to 6. The same technology parameters as the one described above for the comparison of current mirrors were applied. Figure 3-15 shows the current consumption ratio and DC open loop gain difference between the bulk and SOI implementations of the OTA. The FD SOI technology benefits over bulk increase up to a reduction of the supply current by a factor larger than 3.5 and an improvement of the gain by more than 20dB for f_T equal to 10 MHz. As the target transition frequency is increased, the active device g_m/I_D values have to be reduced towards strong inversion, reaching 13 and 3.5 in SOI and bulk respectively at 10MHz.

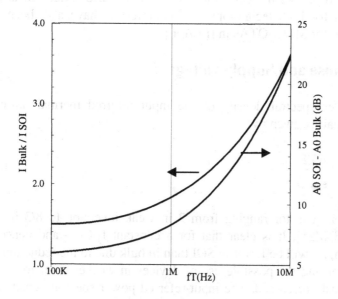

Figure 3-15. Comparison of simulated total current consumption and DC open loop gain of the bulk and SOI cascoded OTAs of Figure 3-14 (with B mirror ratio equal to 2) as a function of the transition frequency. The computations were based on the EKV model. From [SIL96], © 1996 IEEE.

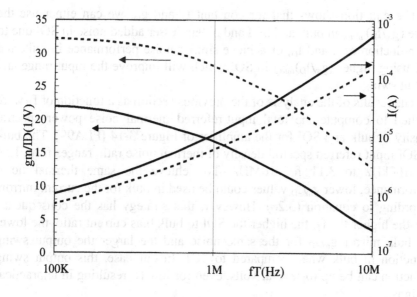

Figure 3-16. Input pair g_m/I_D and current consumption vs. transition frequency for SOI (dashed line) and Bulk (solid line) CMOS OTA. From [SIL96], © 1996 IEEE.

Figure 3-16 shows the g_m/I_D ratio of the input differential pair and total consumption for both technologies. Similar results have also been partly demonstrated for Miller OTAs in [FLA96].

4.2   Noise and Supply voltage

The power spectral density of the input referred thermal noise of a differential pair is given by:

$$S_V = 2 \cdot \frac{\gamma \cdot n \cdot kT}{g_m} \tag{3.25}$$

where γ is a factor ranging from 2 in weak inversion to 8/3 in strong inversion [ENZ95]. It is clear that for a constant $f_T.C_L$ – and hence g_m – specification, S_V will be lower in SOI than in bulk due to the reduction of the n body factor and the possible use of devices in weaker inversion that has been previously discussed. The input-referred power spectral density added by a current mirror is:

$$S_{V,mirror} = 2 \cdot \left(\frac{g_{m,mirror}}{g_m}\right)^2 \cdot \frac{\gamma \cdot n \cdot kT}{g_{m,mirror}} = 2 \cdot \frac{\gamma \cdot n \cdot kT}{g_m^2} \frac{g_{m,mirror}}{I_D} \cdot I_D \tag{3.26}$$

The equation shows that for constant f_T and g_m, we can either use the same $(g_m/I_D)_{mirror}$ in bulk and SOI and obtain lesser added noise in SOI due to the reduction of n and I_D, or achieve similar noise performance in bulk and SOI using higher $(g_m/I_D)_{mirror}$ in SOI which will improve the input range and output swing.

The results of the analysis of the previous section as a function of f_T were applied to compute the total input-referred thermal noise power spectral density in bulk and SOI for the amplifier of Figure 3-14 [FLA99]. The bulk to SOI input referred spectral density of thermal noise ratio ranges from 1.54 for 100kHz to 3.11 for 10MHz. To achieve the same thermal noise performance, lower g_m/I_D values could be used in bulk for the current mirrors according to equation (3.26). However, this strategy has the consequence that the higher the f_T, the higher the SOI to bulk bias current ratio, the lower the bulk mirror g_m/I_D for the same noise and the larger the output swing reduction in bulk when compared to SOI. In our case, this output swing reduction can be up to several volts, even for low f_T, resulting in unpractical designs.

Similar improvements to those computed in the case of the thermal noise are achieved for the 1/f noise characteristics.

The power spectral density of 1/f noise referred to the gate for a single transistor can be modeled as:

$$S_{V,\frac{1}{f}} = \frac{K_F}{C_{ox} WLf} \qquad (3.27)$$

where K_F is a constant that depends on the process and type of transistor (nMOS or pMOS), C_{ox} is the gate oxide capacitance per unit area, W and L the transistor width and length and f the frequency. Measurements results presented in [EGG98] for 1/f noise characteristics of transistors fabricated in the UCL Fully Depleted SOI technology show K_F values very close to those reported for similar Bulk technologies.

Applying for the WL product the expression of Eq. (3.22), we have:

$$S_{V,1/f} = \frac{K_F}{C_{ox}.L^2.g_m} \left(\frac{g_m}{I_D} \right) \left[\frac{I_D}{\left(\frac{W}{L} \right)} \right] \frac{1}{f} \qquad (3.28)$$

Then the 1/f noise power spectral density referred to the input for a differential pair and a current mirror that loads this differential pair (i.e. the equivalent of Eqs. (3.25) and (3.26) in the case of 1/f noise) are given by:

$$S_{V,1/f,diff.p.} = 2 \frac{K_F}{C_{ox}.L^2.g_m.f} \left(\frac{g_m}{I_D} \right) \left[\frac{I_D}{\left(\frac{W}{L} \right)} \right] \qquad (3.29)$$

$$S_{V,1/f,mirror} = 2\frac{K_{F,mirror}}{C_{ox}.L^2_{mirror}.g_m.f}\left(\frac{g_{m,mirror}}{g_m}\right)\left(\left(\frac{g_m}{I_D}\right)\left(\frac{I_D}{\left(\frac{W}{L}\right)}\right)\right)_{mirror} =$$

$$= 2\frac{K_{F,mirror}}{C_{ox}.L^2_{mirror}.g_m.f}\left(\frac{(g_m/I_D)_{mirror}}{(g_m/I_D)}\right)\left(\left(\frac{g_m}{I_D}\right)\left(\frac{I_D}{\left(\frac{W}{L}\right)}\right)\right)_{mirror}$$

(3.30)

In Eq. (3.30) the subscript $_{mirror}$ is used to denote parameters associated to the mirror transistors, while those without subscript correspond to the transistors of the differential pair. The fact that the current through the current mirror and the differential pair transistor are equal was applied to obtain the last expression of Eq. (3.30).

We will now consider the evolution of the input referred 1/f noise spectral density in Bulk and SOI technologies, for a constant transition frequency. As the transition frequency is kept constant, the transconductance of the differential pair, g_m, will be kept constant. The operation in weaker inversion of the SOI amplifier with respect to the Bulk amplifier, leads in SOI to a higher (g_m/I_D) ratio of the differential pair and lower value of the product ((g_m/I_D). $I_D/(W/L)$) (as discussed when we analyzed the current mirror precision, this product decreases in weak inversion because the decrease of $I_D/(W/L)$ in weak inversion is stronger than the increase of (g_m/I_D)). Therefore the 1/f noise contributions of both the differential pair and current mirror will be lower in SOI than in Bulk for equal K_F parameters.

The total input-referred 1/f noise power spectral density in bulk and SOI was computed for the amplifier of Figure 3-14 in bulk and SOI based on the analysis of the previous section as a function of f_T. In the comparison of the previous section, we considered equal g_m/I_D ratios for the current mirrors in the bulk and SOI designs, therefore, the decrease in SOI of the noise contributions of the current mirrors, given by Eq. (3.30), is only due to the higher g_m/I_D ratio of the differential pair, which appears in the denominator. The product ((g_m/I_D). $I_D/(W/L)$) of the mirror, at equal values of the g_m/I_D ratio, is higher in SOI. Nevertheless, the ratio of bulk to SOI total 1/f noise power spectral density ranges, as a function of the OTA specified f_T, from 1 at 100kHz to 2.4 at 10MHz. By exploiting the possibility of having in SOI equal current mirror pole frequency while operating the transistor in weaker inversion, the 1/f noise of the SOI design can be further decreased..

4.3   Offset voltage

The Pelgrom's matching model (Eqs.(3.21)) was applied to compute the offset voltage for the bulk and SOI amplifiers designed in Section 4.1 as a function of the transition frequency. The offset voltage was calculated as follows. Supposing the mismatches of the differential pair and each of the current mirrors of the amplifier of Figure 3-14 are statistically independent, the standard deviation of the offset voltage is given by:

$$\sigma(v_{offset}) = \sqrt{\sigma^2(V_{T0}) + \left(\left(\frac{I_D}{g_m}\right)\frac{\sigma(\beta)}{\beta}\right)^2 + \left(\sigma\left(\frac{\Delta I}{I}\right)_{mirrors}\left(\frac{I_D}{g_m}\right)\right)^2} \qquad (3.31)$$

The first two terms are due to the mismatch of the transistors of the differential pair and the last term is due to the mismatch of the current mirrors. The same notation as above is applied: the terms associated with characteristics of the transistors of the current mirrors are explicitly denoted with a subscript, while those without a subscript correspond to the differential pair transistors. $(\Delta I/I)_{mirrors}$ is the total relative unbalance between the currents of transistors T_3 and T_4 required to compensate the mismatches of mirrors $T_3 - T_5$, $T_4 - T_6$ and $T_7 - T_8$. Based again on the statistically independence of these mismatches, the standard deviation of $(\Delta I/I)_{mirrors}$ can be expressed as a function of these mismatches as:

$$\sigma^2\left(\frac{\Delta I}{I}\right)_{mirrors} = \sigma^2\left(\frac{\Delta I}{I}\right)_{3-5} + \sigma^2\left(\frac{\Delta I}{I}\right)_{4-6} + \sigma^2\left(\frac{\Delta I}{I}\right)_{7-8} \qquad (3.32)$$

The first term, which represents the mismatch of current mirror $T_3 - T_5$, can be directly calculated with Eq. (3.20). In the case of the other two mirrors, they have a current gain B. Considering that the output transistors of these mirrors (T_6 and T_8) are built with B unitary transistors (which is usually the case to improve matching) and that the matching characteristics of these B transistors are statistically independent, we have that:

$$\sigma\left(\frac{\Delta I}{I}\right)_{4,6} = \frac{1}{\sqrt{B}}\sigma\left(\frac{\Delta I}{I}\right)_4 \quad \text{and} \quad \sigma\left(\frac{\Delta I}{I}\right)_{7,8} = \frac{1}{\sqrt{B}}\sigma\left(\frac{\Delta I}{I}\right)_7 \qquad (3.33)$$

where $\sigma(\Delta I/I)_4$ and $\sigma(\Delta I/I)_7$ are determined applying Eq. (3.20) to transistors T_4 and T_7 respectively. This last equation is similar to the well known result, based on properties of the gaussian distribution, that states that the combination of m equal, unitary elements, improves the matching by a square root of m factor.

Consequently, the standard deviation of $(\Delta I/I)_{mirrors}$ is given by:

$$\sigma^2\left(\frac{\Delta I}{I}\right)_{mirrors} = \sigma^2\left(\frac{\Delta I}{I}\right)_3 + \frac{1}{B}\sigma^2\left(\frac{\Delta I}{I}\right)_4 + \frac{1}{B}\sigma^2\left(\frac{\Delta I}{I}\right)_7 \qquad (3.34)$$

The offset voltage is calculated combining Eqs. (3.31) and (3.34) with the expression of $\sigma(\Delta I/I)$ of Eq. (3.20), Pelgrom's matching model of Eq. (3.21) and the data of Table 3-2.

The results are compared in Figure 3-17.

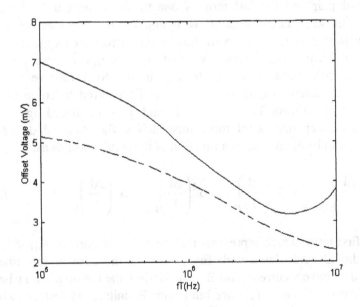

Figure 3-17. Offset voltage vs. transition frequency for SOI (dashed line) and Bulk (solid line) CMOS OTAs.

The offset voltage of these amplifiers is mainly dominated by the effect of the current mirrors mismatch. Since the g_m/I_D ratio of the current mirrors is fixed, as the transition frequency is increased, the current increases and, thus, the transistor W/L aspect ratio increases in order to keep the g_m/I_D ratio constant. This bigger transistors have smaller β and V_{TO} spread, making the offset voltage to decrease as we increase the transition frequency. The increase in offset voltage visible at the higher transition frequency range for the bulk amplifiers is explained because at these frequencies the size of the differential pair transistors drastically decreases in order to reach the low g_m/I_D ratios required, thus increasing the differential pair contribution to the offset voltage. This effect occurs in SOI at higher frequencies.

5.   CONCLUSIONS

This chapter has summarized the characteristics of FD SOI technology relevant for micropower low voltage analog circuits, such as those described in Chapters 1 and 2 for biomedical applications. The analysis of the performance of analog switches showed that in SOI technology an acceptable performance from the point of view of the on-resistance and off current is achievable down to below 1V power supply, while in bulk technologies the minimum supply voltage is around 1.8V. Even for supply voltages that still allow correct operation in bulk, we showed that the speed – accuracy trade off that results from considering the signal dependent charge injection ratio improves in SOI by factors that range from 3 to above 20. A significant increase of the current mirror cut-off frequency and precision is also observed. For OTAs, the characteristics of SOI technology make it possible to achieve current savings that range from 33% up to 70%, with an improvement of the DC gain that goes from 8 to more than 20dB. In bulk designs, the transistors had to be operated closer to strong inversion to achieve the same frequency performance, resulting in a reduction of the input common mode range and output swing, and an increase of the thermal and 1/f noise with regards to FD SOI.

The above analyses were based on the derivation of original mathematical expressions for the estimation of the speed – accuracy trade-off of analog switches as well as the pole frequency and error of current mirrors.

Further comparisons of the performance gains achievable in SOI are shown in Chapters 5 and 6 for experimental prototypes of class AB amplifiers. In Chapter 5 is also discussed, based on the actual layouts of the experimental prototypes, how SOI compares to bulk in terms of die area.

Our work seeks to exploit the superior characteristics of FD SOI technology together with a "power oriented" synthesis methodology and improved circuit architecture. This chapter presented the basis of what is expected at the technological level. Chapter 4 will discuss methodological aspects for power optimization in amplifier design. Chapter 5 will present the novel design approaches applied at the circuit architecture level and finally in Chapter 6 these techniques will join in an experimental demonstration of an ultra low power SOI circuit for a pacemaker sense channel.

Chapter 4

Power Optimization in Operational Amplifier Design

The part of the consumption of a pacemaker that is related to the energy delivered to the heart is below one half of the total consumption. This fraction can be even much smaller depending on the stimulation requirements of the patient. A significant share of the remaining part of the consumption is devoted to the analog circuits that are active most of the time, such as the sense channel or the rate adaptation sensor. The minimization of the consumed power in these circuits is very important in this framework, where savings of even fractions of a μA are significant. This chapter discusses techniques for power optimization in the design of operational amplifiers.

Analog design is characterized by the need to pay attention to multiple performance aspects: bandwidth, gain, noise, slew-rate, input and output voltage ranges, offset .... During the synthesis procedure there are several interactions between these performance aspects, which end up determining the power consumption. This chapter will firstly try to clarify which can be considered the actual root, "independent", main factors that determine power consumption, and which are derived variables. Although the frontiers are not clearly cut and the existence of dependencies among most variables is unavoidable, we think the analysis will help in making clear the general framework for the design procedure. In addition, it will provide comparison criteria for actual implementations.

This analysis will proceed from the general, fundamental aspects to the particular, practical ones. We will start by summarizing current results on the theoretical limits on power consumption of analog circuits. Next, the practical limits will be mentioned and a general scheme will be presented. Finally, we will develop a novel design procedure for the power optimized

85

design of operational amplifiers for a constant total settling time specification.

1.   REVIEW OF THEORETICAL AND PRACTICAL LIMITS ON THE POWER CONSUMPTION OF ANALOG CIRCUITS

1.1   Theoretical limits

The study of the theoretical limits of power consumption of analog circuits has received attention in the last decade, particularly with the contributions and systematization of previous results done by Eric Vittoz [VIT90, VIT95, VIT02]. However, as pointed out by Vittoz in [VIT02], some of the central results had already been proposed nearly 15 years ago [in general in reference HOS85 and for the particular case of switched capacitor filters in reference CAS851].

We will now present what is considered to be the absolute lower boundary for power consumption of analog circuits. This limit is set by the need for achieving a given signal to noise ratio S/N above the lower possible limit of noise associated to thermal noise. The absolute lower boundary for power consumption is achieved in the case of a unity gain low pass filter. In [VIT95, VIT02] this case is first considered and then the case of an amplifier is analyzed. Our derivation will consider the more general situation of a system with gain and the result of unity gain will arise as a particular case.

One important comment on the demonstration of these limits is due here. As stated in [VIT02], there is no rigorous proof that the power calculated through these limits is indeed the minimum possible. Rather, the results are supported on intuition and experience. Nevertheless, the fact that references [VIT95, VIT02 and CAS851] come to the same expressions for circuits based on different principles, (such as continuous time circuits, switched capacitor circuits, and relaxation oscillators), suggests that indeed a more fundamental, physical proof should exist. This is in fact an interesting, open research subject.

The minimum power is derived for the case of an analog module with a load capacitance C, as shown in Figure 4-1 a). This module is considered 100 % efficient, i.e. that all the power coming from the power supply goes to the load capacitance and there is no current consumed internally to the module. We will represent the module through its Norton equivalent model with a transconductance g_m and an output conductance g_o, as shown in Figure 4-1 b). In addition, in Figure 4-1 b) the current source I_N that models the output thermal noise of the module is introduced. This noise current source is characterized by its power spectral density S_I given by:

$$S_I = 4kT\gamma g_m \tag{4.1}$$

where k is the Boltzmann constant, T the absolute temperature, g_m the block transconductance and γ models the noise added by the active circuit implementing the transconductor. γ ranges from 0.5 for a non-degenerated bipolar transistor and $n/2$ for a weakly inverted MOS transistor, where n is the body-effect coefficient or slope factor defined in Chapter 3. In both these cases the resulting transconductance amplifier is strongly nonlinear. When an MOS transistor in strong inversion is considered, γ raises to $(2/3)n$. γ also increases in deep-submicron MOSFETs. A minimum value of $\gamma = 1$ is considered in [VIT95, VIT02].

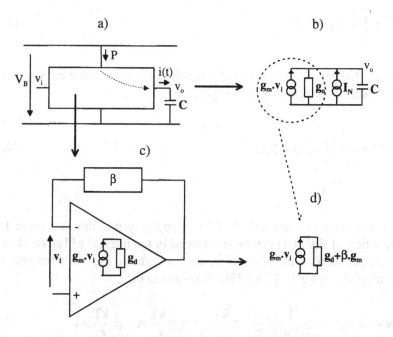

Figure 4-1. Ideal module and model considered for the derivation of the minimum power required for analog signal processing. a) represents the module and related magnitudes: power taken from the power supply P, supply voltage V_B, input and output voltages v_i and v_o, load current $i(t)$ and load capacitance C. b) shows the Norton equivalent model of module a), including the thermal noise current source I_N. c) depicts the particular case when the module a) is implemented with an OTA characterized by its open loop Norton model (with parameters g_m and g_d) and an ideal feedback block with factor β. In d), the resulting closed loop Norton model of the implementation of b) is shown. It results in an output conductance given by $(g_d + \beta \cdot g_m)$.

The consumed power P is derived as follows. If V_{pp} is the peak-to-peak amplitude of the output voltage v_o across C, the average value of the current through C is equal to the signal frequency f multiplied by the charge delivered to C in each cycle: $f.C.V_{pp}$. Then, the average power P delivered from a supply voltage V_B is:

$$P = V_B.f.V_{pp}C = \frac{V_B}{V_{pp}}.f.V_{pp}^2 C \tag{4.2}$$

where in the second expression, V_{pp}^2, which is related to the signal power, is explicitly shown.

The integrated noise power N at the output node v_o can be calculated in the equivalent circuit of Figure 4-1 b) as follows:

$$N = \int_0^{+\infty} S_I.|H(f)|^2 df \tag{4.3}$$

where H(f) represents the transfer function from the noise current source I_N to the output voltage v_o, which is given by:

$$H(s) = \frac{1/g_o}{1 + \frac{s}{g_o/C}}, \quad s = 2.\pi.f \tag{4.4}$$

Either solving the integral of (4.3) or applying that the first order low-pass function of Eq. (4.4) can be substituted in the integral of Eq. (4.3) by an ideal low pass filter with a cut off frequency equal to the –3dB frequency of H(f) multiplied by ($\pi/2$) ([CAR75]), N results to be:

$$N = 4kT\gamma g_m \cdot \frac{1}{g_o^2} \cdot \frac{1}{2\pi} \frac{g_o}{C} \frac{\pi}{2} = \gamma \frac{kT}{C} \frac{g_m}{g_o} = \gamma \frac{kT}{C} A_V \underset{\gamma=1}{\mp} \frac{kT}{C} A_V \tag{4.5}$$

where $A_V = g_m/g_o$ is the low frequency gain of the module.

Applying this expression of the noise power, the signal to noise ratio is given by:

$$\frac{S}{N} = \frac{V_{pp}^2/8}{\frac{kT}{C}A_V} \tag{4.6}$$

Substituting the term $C.V_{pp}^2$ derived from Eq. (4.6) into the expression of the consumed power of Eq. (4.2) we have:

$$P = \frac{V_B}{V_{pp}}f.8kTA_V \frac{S}{N} \tag{4.7}$$

The factor $V_B.A_V/V_{pp}$ is always greater or equal than 1. This is so because if A_V is greater or equal than one, then the supply voltage V_B must be greater than (or, in an ideal limit case, equal to) the output peak to peak voltage V_{pp}[2]. If A_V is less than one, the minimum supply voltage is determined by the input peak to peak voltage, then:

$$V_B \geq V_{ipp} = \frac{V_{pp}}{A_V} => \frac{V_B}{V_{pp}}A_V \geq 1 \tag{4.8}$$

Then the absolute minimum is reached when $A_V=1$ and $V_B = V_{pp}$ or $A_V < 1$ and $V_B = V_{ipp} = V_{pp}/A_V$, in these cases:

$$P_{min} = 8kTf \frac{S}{N}, \quad A_V : 1 \tag{4.9}$$

If the circuit provides a gain A_V greater than 1, then:

$$P_{min} = 8kTf \frac{S}{N}.A_V, \quad A_V > 1 \tag{4.10}$$

In these equations, f represents the circuit bandwidth, considering the S/N value is required up to the maximum bandwidth frequency.

The same result is obtained if we consider that the block of Figure 4-1 a) is implemented as a closed loop amplifier as shown in Figure 4-1 c). In this case, as shown in Figure 4-1 d), the resulting output conductance g_o is given by:

---

[2] An exception are the circuits in fully diferential or "bridge" configuration. In these cases the minimum supply voltage is equal to half the peak to peak output voltage. In this case the right half of Eq. (4.7) is divided by 2 and the minimum power given by Eq. (4.10) is divided by 4.

$$g_o = g_d + \beta \cdot g_m \Rightarrow A_V = \frac{g_m}{g_o} = \frac{g_m/g_d}{1 + \left(g_m/g_d\right)\beta} \qquad (4.11)$$

Therefore the same expressions results substituting A_V by the closed loop gain of the amplifier of Figure 4-1 c).

Some interesting consequences are derived from Eqs. (4.7) to (4.9).

- Eq. (4.7) shows the importance of approaching rail to rail operation in order to minimize the factor V_B/V_{pp}.
- The minimum value of Eq. (4.9) shows the theoretical minimum power consumption has strong dependence with S/N, gain and bandwidth (through the f factor).

In reference [VIT02], it is shown that the minimum given by Eq. (4.8) holds for relaxation oscillators and that the implementation of high quality factor (Q) poles through active resonators (without inductors) leads to an increase of the minimum power required by a factor $4.Q^2$.

1.2   Practical limits

Several elements add to the baseline set by the thermal noise in order to determine the total power consumption in practical circuits. A summary of these elements, whose effects are discussed in detail in [VIT02], follows.

- *Parasitic capacitors.* They demand increased g_m, and hence current, to reach the required speed. In op amps, parasitic capacitors introduce a phase shift leading to the use of a compensating capacitor that increases the current required to reach a given gain-bandwidth product.
- *Additional sources of noise.* Any unwanted signal falling inside the circuit bandwidth is included in this group. Examples of these noise sources are: flicker noise (1/f), interfering signals which require higher CMRR (common mode signals) or higher PSRR (interference through the power supply lines) or higher linearity (interference due to intermodulation products of out of band signals) and charge injection of switches. These noise sources increase the power in two ways. Either an increase of the signal power is required to maintain the signal-to-noise ratio or changes in the circuit structures are required to decrease the effect of these noise sources. Examples of these circuit changes are the use of bigger devices, which introduce bigger parasitic capacitances, to reduce 1/f noise; the application of more complex and power hungry circuits that improve CMRR or PSRR, or the increase in the linear range of transconductors, which is associated with a decrease in the g_m/I_D ratio.

- **Mismatch of components.** Matching of components is a fundamental analog design tool that is required to be independent of parasitic effects and process variations. In order to improve matching, bigger components are required, which results in increased parasitic capacitances and power.
- **Non optimum supply voltage.** As discussed above the most efficient situation takes place when the supply voltage is just the minimum required to accommodate the circuit voltage swings. Reductions of the voltage swing, such as those due to the transistors' saturation and gate-source or base-emitter voltages, result in an increase of power.
- **Non linear circuit behavior.** The theoretical analysis of the previous section assumed a system that is perfectly linear. However, practical circuit structures and actual device characteristics are inherently non linear. Consequently, non linear effects are always present to some extent. Examples of these effects are harmonic distortion due to the non linear characteristics of devices and slew rate limitation in differential pairs and class A output stages. These effects must be limited and to do so means increased power. This increase in power may come, for example, from the utilization of reduced ratios of voltage or current signal amplitude to bias levels in order to limit harmonic distortion or from an increase in bias current to rise the slew rate limits.

In the next section we will consider how these general considerations apply in a particular circuit (Miller OTA) and show a way to optimize the speed – power trade-off in this case.

1.3 Figures of Merit for the Power Efficiency of Analog Circuits.

The theoretical limit discussed above gives way to a first figure of merit for analog circuits, from the point of view of the power efficiency. It stems from Eq. (4.9), and is given by: ([VIT02])

$$K = \frac{P}{k.T.\Delta f.\frac{S}{N}} \tag{4.12}$$

According to the previous results, K has a minimum value of 8.

Alternatively, simplified versions of this figure of merit have been applied to operational amplifiers and filters in order to represent the frequency–power tradeoff. In reference [ESC95] the gain-bandwidth divided by the consumed power is applied (GHz/W) and in [NG99], the load capacitance is taken into account in the trade-off and the ratio of power to gain-bandwidth multiplied by the load capacitance (mW/MHz.pF) is applied.

Reference [KRI01] compares filters based on the power divided by bandwidth and order of the filter, and this figure of merit is plotted against the input range of each filter, resulting in a similar comparison to that of Eq. (4.12).

As shown in Eq. (4.10), when an amplifier is considered, its gain must also be taken into account in the comparison.

2. OPERATIONAL AMPLIFIER POWER OPTIMIZATION FOR A GIVEN TOTAL (SLEWING PLUS LINEAR) SETTLING TIME

The analyses presented in the previous section identify noise, speed (signal frequency) and voltage gain as the ultimate factors setting the minimum power consumption of amplifiers.

Table 4-1 shows, for the case of an operational amplifier, a hierarchical representation intended to serve as a general guideline on how these factors relate to the amplifier specifications and to lower level design aspects.

Table 4-1. Hierarchical representation of the main factors that determine power consumption in operational amplifiers.

High Level Performance Data	Medium Level Performance Data	Low Level Data
Speed or Dynamic Precision (Total Settling Time, Frequency)	Linear Settling Time (transition frequency, phase margin)	Transconductances, Currents, (W/L), Compensation Capacitance
	Slew Rate	Currents, Compensation or Load Capacitance
Signal to Noise Ratio, Noise	Voltage Swings, Supply Voltage	Currents, (W/L)
	Thermal Noise	Transconductances, Compensation Capacitance
	1/f Noise	Transconductances, W, L
Static Precision	DC Gain	Transconductances, Currents, L
	Offset Voltage	Transconductances, Currents

From left to right, the minimum power consumption required is conditioned by what is demanded at the amplifier overall performance level, which we have referred to as "high level performance data". This high level data is represented by the ability of the amplifier to follow fast input signals (i.e. speed, dynamic precision, which in the case of the following study is represented by the total settling time), by the total noise and by the static precision, i.e. the output error with DC inputs. The high level data, which is the significant one at the system level, is determined by "medium level" performance of the amplifier, where more than one mechanism combine to determine each high-level performance data. Finally, each "medium level" characteristic of the amplifier can be correlated to the "low level" design details: the transistors' transconductance and current (which determine the (W/L) aspect ratio as shown in [SIL96]), as well as the compensation capacitance and transistors' length.

In the conventional, current, design practice, the step that goes from the high-level performance data to the medium level performance data that guides amplifier design, has been based on rather fuzzy rules. This is particularly noticeable in the case of the total settling time. In addition, power consumption usually has been a secondary output of the design procedure. In this section, we propose a new approach to transit systematically from the high level total settling time specification to a low-level design that complies with this specification with optimum power consumption. This approach is based on the g_m/I_D methodology [SIL96] that allows a systematic exploration of the design space to implement the step that goes from the medium level op amp specifications to the low level design data.

We will particularly focus on the first row of Table 4-1, which addresses the settling behavior of amplifiers. The other specifications will be checked a posteriori for the power-optimized design and the initial selection of parameters (transistor lengths, compensation capacitor) for the design would be changed if these other specifications were not met.

The settling behavior is an essential specification in most op amp applications, particularly A/D and D/A converters and sampled data filters. It is a direct measure of the ability of the amplifier to respond to large input signals [CHU82]. The total settling time is defined as the time the response to an input step will take to settle to a given relative error (e.g. 1 %) of its final value.

Two distinct periods determine the settling time: the slewing period and the linear settling period.

During the slewing period, the variation rate of the output is limited to a maximum value (slew rate). This originates from the charging of a capacitive node with a limited, constant current. This node can be either an internal node (e.g. the first stage output node in a Miller amplifier) or, particularly in the case of class A operational transconductance amplifiers (OTAs), the output node. We will refer to the first case as internal slew rate and to the second one as external slew rate.

The second part of the settling time is the linear settling period, for which the amplifier behaves linearly, according to its small signal frequency response. The linear settling time is related to the amplifier transition frequency and phase margin.

Researchers have devoted attention for a long time to the issue of settling time modeling in operational amplifiers [KAM74, CHU82, TUR83, LIN86, WAN95]. In [KAM74] the influence of pole-zero doublets was first pointed-out and some initial modeling of slew rate and settling time was presented. Reference [CHU82] introduces a model considering the slew rate effect and a second order small signal frequency response for the amplifier. In [TUR83] and [LIN86], the model in [CHU82] is completed by considering the initial condition on the derivative of voltage with respect to time, for the analysis of the linear part of settling. This derivative is supposed to be zero in [CHU82]. Finally, in [WAN95] the classical approximation for slew rate is improved through a large signal analysis of the output stage during the input stage slewing period. However, this analysis considers the particular case of a square-law, strong inversion, equation for the active transistor of the output stage.

Contrasting with this analysis effort, almost no antecedent is found that systematically addresses the issue from a synthesis perspective. For synthesis purposes, in many applications, the significant parameter is the total settling time. A given total settling time can be achieved with different distributions between the linear settling and the slewing part. Which is the best alternative to this distribution is still unresolved. For example, in the switched capacitor domain, usually the slewing period is assigned an arbitrary part of the available time for settling (10% is taken as an example in p. 497 of [GRE86] and in [TAY94] a 25% allotment to slew rate is suggested).

As we show in this work, the selected partition strongly influences power consumption ([SIL022]). Therefore, we have tried to answer the following question:

Which is the best combination, in terms of consumption, between slew rate and gain bandwidth product for a given total settling time in the response to a step of given amplitude?

Regarding the design and applying the g_m/I_D methodology [SIL96], we discuss the following question:

How does the answer to the above question impact on the design decisions in the synthesis of an operational amplifier? Particularly, how does it affect the selection of the g_m/I_D ratios or inversion levels for the active transistors of the amplifier?

The section is organized as follows. First, we present the model of settling behavior applied for our synthesis. The model is checked against experimental measurements. The design equations and synthesis procedure are then introduced. Subsection 2.3 presents the results of applying a complete design space exploration in a non-simplified case. Simulation results that validate the proposed methodology are also included in this subsection. Finally the resulting optimum designs are compared in Bulk and SOI technologies.

2.1   Design Oriented Model of Settling Behavior

Our objective is to have an expression of the total settling time suitable to be applied in an analytical synthesis procedure and in qualitative hand analysis. This goal discourages the application of the more exact, but very complex, expressions that result when a second order model is considered for the amplifier as in [CHU82, TUR83, LIN86, WAN95].

We will apply a first order model of the amplifier in order to determine the basic expression of total settling time. The fact that the actual system has higher order terms alters both the linear settling and the slewing periods. The change in the linear settling time due to effect of the higher order terms, as shown in ([LAK94],p. 626), is not important when the phase margin is between 60 and 70 degrees. In addition, we will consider it by adjusting the number of time constants required for settling with a given precision. In order to include the effect of a second order system on the slewing period with more precision, the analysis must take into account that slew rate is not a small signal phenomenon and thus, perform a non linear analysis of the second stage (when the slew rate originates in the first stage), as discussed in [WAN95]. This increases even more the model complexity. This added complexity, besides jeopardizing our goal of having a tractable expression for design, might not reach its aim of increased precision if other effects that affect the actual value of slew rate (which are not considered in [WAN95]) are not taken into account. One of these effects is the influence on the input stage slew rate of the parasitic capacitance that is in parallel with the differential pair tail current source. An additional drawback is that the more detailed the model, the more it becomes linked to particularities of a given amplifier architecture. The model we will apply has a reasonable accuracy, which allows us to take design decisions, while it is independent from the amplifier architecture and considers the effect of both the internal and external slew rates. This last feature is a further advantage over previous complex models [CHU82, TUR83, LIN86, WAN95] that only take the internal slew rate into account.

Our model, shown in Figure 4-2, considers the amplifier in a closed loop with a real feedback factor β.

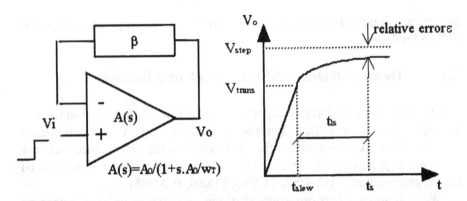

Figure 4-2. Model for total settling time analysis. The amplifier is modeled with an open loop DC gain A_0, transition frequency $w_T/(2.\pi)$ and a real feedback factor β. The plot of the output voltage vs. time shows the slewing period (t_{slew}), the linear settling (t_{ls}), the total settling time (t_s) and the output voltage where the transition from the slew rate limited operation to linear operation occurs (V_{trans}). From [SIL022], © 2002 IEEE.

When the amplifier operates linearly, supposing the open loop A_0 is much larger than $(1/\beta)$, the closed loop low frequency gain is $1/\beta$ and the time constant τ is given by:

$$\tau = \frac{1}{\beta.w_T} \tag{4.13}$$

with w_T the transition angular frequency.

The step response of this first order system from an initial value of V_{init} to a final value V_f is given by:

$$V_o = (V_f - V_{init}).(1 - e^{-\frac{t}{\tau}}) + V_{init} \tag{4.14}$$

Its slope is maximum at t=0, and is given by:

$$\left. \frac{dV_o}{dt} \right|_{max} = \frac{(V_f - V_{init})}{\tau} \tag{4.15}$$

The transition between the slew rate limited region and linear operation happens when the current demanded, assuming linear operation, by the stage that is in slew-rate falls just below the maximum value that sets the slew-rate. When a first order model is considered for the amplifier, since the second stage is acting with a frequency independent gain, it can be shown that this transition occurs when the slope imposed at the output by the amplifier dynamics, which is given in the last equation, is equal to the slew rate. This result applies both for the internal and external slew-rates. In the case of the internal slew-rate it coincides with the result from analyzing which is the input voltage that makes the output current of the first stage to saturate. Therefore, by considering a first order model for the amplifier we manage to treat jointly the case of the internal and external slew-rates.

Applying this criterium, the output voltage when the transition occurs (V_{trans} in Figure 4-2), verifies:

$$\frac{(V_{step} - V_{trans})}{\tau} = SR \qquad (4.16)$$

with $V_f = V_{step}$ the amplitude of the output step, which is equal to the input step divided by β.

The slew rate dominated part of the total settling (t_{slew} in Figure 4-2) is given by:

$$t_{slew} = \begin{cases} \dfrac{V_{trans}}{SR} = \dfrac{V_{step} - \tau.SR}{SR} = \dfrac{V_{step}}{SR} - \tau \ (V_{step} > \tau.SR) \\ 0 \ (V_{step} \leq \tau.SR) \end{cases} \qquad (4.17)$$

The linear settling time, t_{ls} in Figure 4-2, defined as the time it takes the output to settle to V_{step} with a relative error less than ε, and taking into account that the initial condition is V_{trans}, is given by:

$$t_{ls} = t / \frac{|V_o - V_{step}|}{V_{step}} = \varepsilon \Rightarrow t_{ls} = \tau.\left(\ln\left(\tfrac{1}{\varepsilon}\right) + \ln\left(\frac{\tau.SR}{V_{step}} \right) \right) \qquad (4.18)$$

where t is time and V_o the output voltage.

This expression for the linear settling time has two terms. The first one ($\tau.\ln(1/\varepsilon)$) is the usual approximation for the linear settling time. It is the settling time to relative error ε of a first order system with time constant τ. However, when we take into account the slewing part of the step response, the step amplitude in the linear part becomes smaller than the total step. We have ($V_{step} - V_{trans}$) instead of V_{step}. Therefore, the time required to reach the final value with a given relative error ε with respect to the total step amplitude V_{step} is smaller than ($\tau.\ln(1/\varepsilon)$). The second term is indeed negative since the argument of the logarithm is always less than one (it is equal to $(V_{step} - V_{trans})/V_{step}$).

The expression of the total settling time, taking into account the slewing and the linear part, is given by:

$$t_s = t_{ls} + t_{slew} = \tau \left[\ln\left(\tfrac{1}{\varepsilon}\right) - 1 + \ln\left(\frac{\tau.SR}{V_{step}} \right) + \frac{V_{step}}{\tau.SR} \right] = \tau \left[\ln\left(\tfrac{1}{\varepsilon}\right) - 1 + \ln(x) + \frac{1}{x} \right]$$

$$(4.19)$$

where x is a dimensionless magnitude equal to $\tau.SR/V_{step}$. From (4.16) we have that

$$x = \frac{\tau.SR}{V_{step}} = \frac{V_{step} - V_{trans}}{V_{step}} \qquad\qquad (4.20)$$

Therefore x takes values between 0 and 1, and its physical meaning is that it corresponds to the fraction of the total step where we have linear settling.

The expression (4.19) of the total settling time evaluates to $(\tau \ln(1/\varepsilon))$ at x=1. In this case, there is no slewing part, only linear settling. Then, we have as result the settling time of the linear system.

(4.19) tends to infinity when x tends to 0. For a given V_{step}, x tending to 0 means either τ tends to 0 or SR tends to 0. In both cases the number of time constants τ required for settling tends to infinity, either because τ tends to 0 for a finite SR or because SR tends to 0 for a finite τ.

The following figures show the evolution with x, of the following characteristics of the amplifier settling behavior: the total settling time t_s over the small signal time constant τ (Figure 4-3), the fraction of the total settling time dominated by the slew rate ((t_{slew}/t_s), Figure 4-4, solid line) and the fraction with linear operation ((t_{ls}/t_s), Figure 4-4, dashed line). In Figure 4-3 the cases of 1% and 0.1% relative error are considered, while in Figure 4-4 the case of 1% relative error is considered. It is interesting to note that these curves depend only on the required precision (ε).

In Figure 4-3 we can see that for x equal to 1 and 1% relative error, we have t_s equal to 4.6 τ, which is equal to $\ln(1/\varepsilon)$ with the considered value of ε equal to 0.01 (1% relative error). For x equal to 0.1, i.e. 90% of the output voltage transient in slew rate mode, we have that the number of time constants required for settling rise to about 11. This figure therefore give us a first idea, on how the partition of the total transient between the slew rate limited mode and the linear mode affects the total time required.

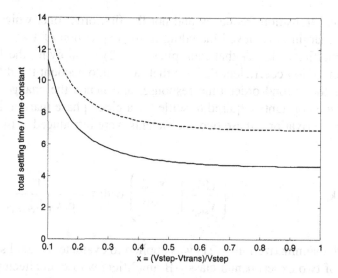

Figure 4-3. Total settling time over time constant as a function of x (fraction of voltage step in linear operation) for 1% relative error (solid line) and 0.1% relative error (dashed line).

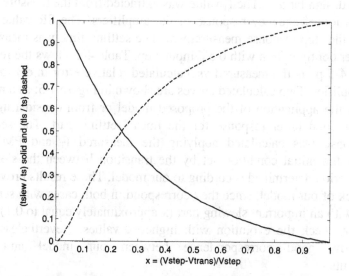

Figure 4-4. Fraction of the total settling time dominated by the slew rate ((tslew/ts), solid line) and the fraction with linear operation ((tls/ts), dashed line) as a function of x (fraction of voltage step in linear operation) for 1% relative error.

The fact that the amplifier has actually a second order response, can be taken into account by introducing two changes to (4.19): (1) calculating τ

with the actual transition frequency and not the first order one, which for a given phase margin is achieved including in the expression of τ of (4.13) a correction coefficient k_{corrwT} that multiplies w_T; (2) multiplying the $\ln(1/\varepsilon)$ term by a correction coefficient ($k_{corrsetl}$) that takes into account the different evolution of the second order time response, and hence the change in the number of time constants required to settle for a given phase margin. For all the following derivations, these two coefficients were introduced in (4.19) as follows:

$$t_s = \tau \left(k_{corrsetl} \ln\left(\tfrac{1}{\varepsilon}\right) - 1 + \ln\left(\frac{\tau.SR}{V_{step}}\right) + \frac{V_{step}}{\tau.SR} \right) \text{ with } \tau = \frac{1}{\beta.w_T.k_{corrwT}} \quad (4.21)$$

The model summarized in (4.21) was applied to evaluate the total settling time at 5% of two experimental class AB amplifiers whose architecture will be described in Chapter 5. These are a 9MHz class AB OTA in a 0.8μm Bulk CMOS technology and a 5.6MHz class AB OTA in a 2μm FD SOI technology. Since the goal of this evaluation is to check the settling time model against experimental results, we used the measured f_T and SR values and not the design targets. The f_T value was extracted from the measurement of the open loop frequency response of the amplifiers. The SR value was taken from the step response measurement. The settling time was measured in a follower configuration with 0.5V input step. Table 4-2 shows the results and Figure 4-5 plots the measured vs. calculated relative error in dB for the FD SOI amplifier. Two calculated curves are shown in Figure 4-5: as a result either from the application of the proposed model or from considering the calculated second order response for the linear settling part. The second order response was calculated applying the measured f_T and PM and considering the initial condition set by the transition between the slewing and linear period determined according to our model. These results provide a partial check of our model, since they correspond in both cases with settling behaviors with an important slewing part (x approximately equal to 0.1), and thus do not check the evolution with higher x values. Nevertheless, the results show good correspondence between our model and the measurements.

Table 4-2. Comparison of calculated and measured total settling time at 5% error with a 0.5V input step for two class AB OTAs in follower configuration. The value applied for the correction factor $k_{corrsetl}$ is shown. The correction factor k_{corrwT} was not applied; the actual w_T value (not the first order one) was applied instead.

Technology	f_T (MHz)	PM (°)	SR(V/μs)	t_s measured (ns)	t_s calculated (ns)	$k_{corrsetl}$
Bulk	9.0	57	3.2	157	169	1.3
FD SOI	5.6	64	1.6	311	305	1.05

2.2   Power Optimization of a Miller OTA for Given Total Settling Time.

Without any loss of generality, we will develop our power optimization methodology based on the case of the RC compensated Miller OTA shown in Figure 4-6. We have chosen the RC compensation because it allows us to eliminate the right half plane zero of Miller compensation, thus reducing the requirements on the second stage transconductance and making it possible to reduce the power consumption. The RC compensation introduces an additional non-dominant pole, but it can be shown to lie at much higher frequencies than the first non-dominant pole, associated to the load capacitance.

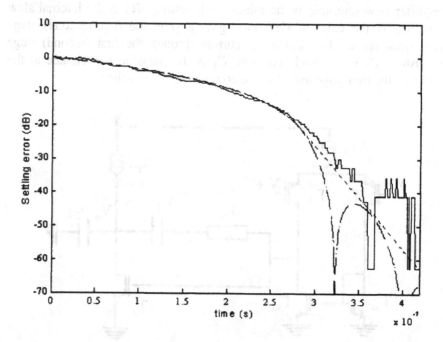

Figure 4-5. Relative settling error in dB for a 5.6MHz FD SOI, class AB amplifier. Measurement (solid line), calculated with the proposed model (short dashes line), and calculated with second order model for linear settling (long dashes line).

The following equations summarize the relationships between the Miller amplifier characteristics and the "low level" design parameters that we will need to formulate our design procedure [LAK94]:

$$f_{TI} = \frac{1}{2\pi} \frac{g_{ml}}{C_f} \qquad (4.22)$$

$$PM = f(f_{T1}, f_{ndp}) \text{ with } f_{T1} = \frac{1}{2\pi} \frac{g_{m1}}{C_f} \text{ and } f_{ndp} = \frac{1}{2\pi} \frac{g_{m2}.C_f}{C_1 C_2 + C_f(C_1 + C_2)}$$

$$\Rightarrow f_{ndp} = k.f_{T1} \text{ to assure given phase margin (PM)}, k = 2.2 \text{ for } PM = 67°$$

$$(4.23)$$

$$SR = \min(SR_1, SR_2), \text{ with } SR_1 = \frac{2.I_{D1}}{C_f} \text{ and } SR_2 = \frac{I_{D2}}{C_2} \qquad (4.24)$$

where PM is the phase margin, f_{T1} is the first order unity-gain or transition frequency, f_{ndp} is the non dominant pole frequency, SR is the total amplifier slew rate, min is the minimum function, SR1 is the internal slew rate, SR_2 is the external slew rate, g_{m1} (g_{m2}) is the first (second) stage transconductance, I_{D1} (I_{D2}) is the current through the first (second) stage transistors, C_2 is the load capacitor, C_1 is the parasitic capacitance at the output of the first stage and C_f is the compensation capacitor.

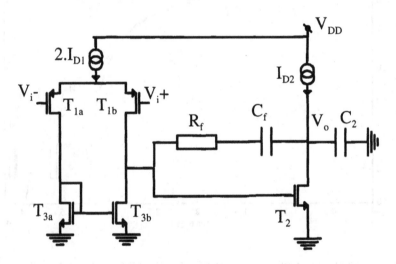

Figure 4-6.. RC compensated Miller OTA applied to develop power optimization methodology.

An additional equation is related to the determination of the compensation capacitor. This can be done in two ways.

The first lies in the fact that the compensation capacitor determines the thermal noise characteristic of the amplifier ([LAK94], pp. 523 to 535). The total equivalent integrated white noise at the input in a –3dB bandwidth of f_T

(which is the case for a follower connected amplifier), provided that the output stage contribution is negligible, is given by:

$$v_{inw} = \sqrt{2\left(1 + \frac{g_{m3}}{g_{m1}}\right)\frac{2}{3}\cdot\frac{kT}{C_f}}$$ (4.25)

where g_{m1} and g_{m3} are respectively the transconductances of the input differential pair and input stage current mirror transistors. The range of variation of the ratio (g_{m3}/g_{m1}) is not very wide because both transistors have the same bias current so that:

$$\frac{g_{m3}}{g_{m1}} = \frac{\left(g_m/I_D\right)_3}{\left(g_m/I_D\right)_1}$$ (4.26)

This ratio will usually vary at most in a range of about ¼ to 4, and in most cases in a smaller range[3]. Therefore, *the equivalent input voltage due to white noise is mainly determined by the value of the compensating capacitance C_f.*

Consequently, a first way is to determine C_f from the noise specification. A second way to determine C_f is from the effect it has on power consumption. If we consider a given transition frequency, Eq. (4.22) shows that an increase in C_f requires an increase in the first stage transconductance and thus an increase in the first stage current. On the other hand, for a given phase margin and thus a given non dominant pole frequency, from Eq. (4.23) it can be seen that an increase in C_f results in a decrease in the necessary g_{m2} and hence a decrease in the second stage current. Therefore there is an optimum C_f value that results in a minimum total current, for a given transition frequency and phase margin.

We will consider that either C_f is deduced from the noise specification or it is determined during the design procedure to give the minimum power consumption.

Finally Eq. (4.21) gives the total settling time as a function of f_{T1} and SR:

---

[3] In low-power/low-voltage applications, the transistors are not biased deep in strong inversion, hence reducing the spread of values of the g_m/I_D ratio that will be applied.

$$t_s = f(f_{T1}, SR) = \tau \cdot \left(k_{corrsetl} \ln\left(\tfrac{1}{\varepsilon}\right) - 1 + \ln\left(\frac{\tau . SR}{V_{step}}\right) + \frac{V_{step}}{\tau . SR} \right)$$

(4.27)

with $\tau = \dfrac{1}{\beta . 2 . \pi . f_{T1} . k_{corrwT}}$

Considering the previous equations, we have five unknowns and three equations. The five unknowns are: the (W/L) and currents of the input and output transistors and the compensation capacitance, or equivalently: g_m/I_D of the input and output transistors, f_{T1}, current of the output transistor (I_{D2}) and compensation capacitance (C_f). The equations are Eq. (4.23) to have a given phase margin, Eq. (4.27) to have a given total settling time and the condition that determines the compensation capacitance (any among the two presented alternatives). Hence, we have two degrees of freedom that we will assign to the g_m/I_D ratios of the input differential pair transistors (($g_m/I_D)_1$) and of the output stage active transistor (($g_m/I_D)_2$). Our goal will be to determine the combination of ($g_m/I_D)_1$ and ($g_m/I_D)_2$ that results in minimum power consumption.

The design procedure explores the design space as follows:

1   The lengths of the active transistors are initially taken at minimum value. This value can be later increased in order to improve other performance aspects such as DC gain, 1/f noise characteristic, matching or offset.

2   A value is chosen for the g_m/I_D ratio of the input stage current mirror transistors (which we will refer to as T_{3a} and T_{3b}). The ratio $I_{D1}/(W/L)_3$ is deduced from the g_m/I_D vs. $I_D/(W/L)$ curve ([SIL96]). Then $(W/L)_3$ is calculated, since the current through $T_{3a,b}$ is equal to the current through the differential pair transistors (I_{D1}). ($g_m/I_D)_3$ can be later adjusted if the pole of the current mirror lies too close to the amplifier bandwith.

3   The design space is explored by systematically sweeping the parameters: ($g_m/I_D)_1$, ($g_m/I_D)_2$, and C_f (this last one, in case it is not fixed from the noise specification). For each combination of these parameters, the amplifier is designed to comply with the total settling time specified and to have a given phase margin. This is done by the following iterative procedure:

3.1   Initial values are determined for f_{T1} and I_{D2}. This can be done by solving Eqs. (4.13) to (4.27) in the simplified case where $C_1 \ll C_f \ll C_2$ and $I_{D2} \gg I_{D1}$.

3.2 I_{D1} is determined as:

$$I_{D1} = \frac{2\pi f_{T1} C_f}{\left(\frac{g_m}{I_D}\right)_1} \tag{4.28}$$

3.3 Since now the (g_m/I_D) ratios and currents are known for all the transistors $T_1..T_3$, (W/L) and then W and L are determined applying the relationship between g_m/I_D and $(I_D/(W/L))$ ([SIL96]).

$$\left(\frac{g_m}{I_D}\right) \Rightarrow \left(\frac{I_D}{\left(\frac{W}{L}\right)}\right) \Rightarrow \left(\frac{W}{L}\right) = \frac{I_D}{\left(\frac{I_D}{\left(\frac{W}{L}\right)}\right)} \tag{4.29}$$

3.4 From the calculated transistor sizes, the parasitic capacitance C_1 is calculated and then the parameter x defined in section 2.1, f_{T1} and I_{D2} are recalculated with the following equations that are derived from Eqs. (4.19) to (4.24) and (4.27).

$$I_{D2} = 2\pi f_{T1} \frac{2.2(C_1 C_2 - C_f (C_1 - C_2))}{\left(\frac{g_m}{I_D}\right)_2 C_f}$$

$$x = \frac{\min\left[\frac{2}{\left(\frac{g_m}{I_D}\right)_1}, \frac{2.2(C_1 C_2 + C_f (C_1 + C_2))}{\left(\frac{g_m}{I_D}\right)_2 C_f C_2}\right]}{\beta.k_{corrwT}.V_{step}} \Rightarrow$$

$$\Rightarrow f_{T1} = \frac{\left(k_{corrsetl}.\ln\left(\frac{1}{\varepsilon}\right) - 1 + \ln(x) + \frac{1}{x}\right)}{2.\pi.\beta.k_{corrwT}.t_s} \tag{4.30}$$

3.5 If the relative difference with the initial values of f_{T1} and I_{D2} is less than a given error then the procedure is finished, otherwise we iterate at step 3.2 with the calculated values of f_{T1} and I_{D2}.

This procedure only calculates the dimensions of the active transistors $T_1...T_3$, the transistors of the current sources can be later sized for the selected optimum design, since their size does not influence the settling time to the first order.

An interesting feature of the proposed procedure is that, though it is developed in the case of a Miller RC compensated OTA, it can be very easily applied to other architectures. This is based on the following considerations.

a) As discussed above, the total settling time model is fairly independent of the particular amplifier architecture.

b) The most general concept of exploring the design space through the g_m/I_D method to search for the minimum consumption for a given total settling time, can be, of course, applied to any amplifier. What is needed are suitable set of equations and design procedure based on the g_m/I_D methodology for this amplifier

c) The particular design procedure that we have just described for the Miller RC amplifier, which tells us how to iterate to find the solution, can be also extended to other cases. This procedure is based on the two expressions given in Eq. (4.23) that relate the first order transition frequency with the input stage g_m/I_D ratio and the non dominant pole with the output stage g_m/I_D ratio. These same dependencies are present in other amplifiers. This is for example the case of the folded cascode OTA, considering as $(g_m/I_D)_2$ the g_m/I_D ratio of the cascode transistors.

2.3   Results of Complete Design Space Exploration and Comparison with Simulation Results

The procedure described in the previous paragraph was applied to the design of a Miller OTA in the 3µm CMOS on FD SOI technology of Université catholique de Louvain, Belgium ([FLA01]). The design specifications are a total 1% settling time of 1µs for an input step of amplitude V_{step} equal to 0.25V and a 10 pF load capacitor, typical for operational amplifiers for instrumentation. The active transistors' lengths were taken equal to the minimum value (3µm) and the (g_m/I_D) ratio of the current mirror was taken equal to 10.

An exploration of the design space as described above, gave as result that the value of the compensating capacitor that minimizes the total current consumption is 2pF. Figure 4-7 shows the variation of the minimum total current as a function of the compensation capacitance. In Figure 4-8, C_f was taken fixed at the optimum value of 2pF and the curves with constant consumption in the plane $(g_m/I_D)_1$, $(g_m/I_D)_2$ are shown.

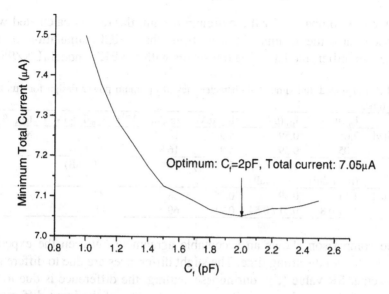

Figure 4-7. Minimum total current as a function of the compensation capacitor C_f for a Miller OTA in a 3μm CMOS on FD SOI technology with 1μs total 1% settling time with a 0.25V step on a 10pF load.

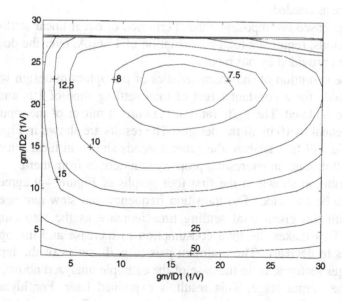

Figure 4-8. Constant total current consumption as a function of input and output stages (g_m/I_D) ratios for a given 1μs total settling time. From [SIL022], © 2002 IEEE.

Table 4-3 compares, for the optimum design, the results calculated with our model and the results obtained from the SPICE simulation of the designed amplifier, modeling the transistors with the EKV model [ENZ95].

Table 4-3. Calculated and simulated characteristics of optimum power design for 1µs total settling time.

	I_{tot} (µA)	I_{D1} (µA)	I_{D2} (µA)	$(g_m/I_D)_1$ (V^{-1})	$(g_m/I_D)_2$ (V^{-1})	t_{ls}/t_s (%)
Calculated	7.05	0.59	5.9	16	23	80
SPICE	7.05	0.59	5.9	16.8	24.4	-
	ts (µs) (rise / fall)	SR (V/µs) (rise / fall)	ft (MHz)	PM (°)	AO (dB)	
Calculated	1 / 1	0.59	0.75	68	82	
SPICE	1.2 / 0.8	0.41 / 0.54	0.71	69	88	

The comparison shows an acceptable agreement between the expected values for the total settling time. The slight differences are due to differences in the actual SR value (e.g. during rise settling, the difference is due to the influence of the parasitic capacitance at the sources of the input differential pair) and to variations in the linear settling due to the fact that the output transistor does not really operate in a small signal way during the transient. Nevertheless, the achieved agreement validates the application of the method in order to determine an initial design that can be fine tuned for the desired performance as needed.

A design based on imposing a usual criterion of equal linear settling and slewing periods, requires a total consumption of 15.6µA, over the double of the optimum provided by our method.

Next the evolution of the characteristics of the optimum design with the step amplitude for a constant target of total settling time of 1µs and 10pF load were calculated. The g_m/I_D ratio of the current mirror of the input stage was taken equal to 10 in all the designs. The results are shown in Figure 4-9 a) to e). We will first analyze the general trends shown in these curves and then we will discuss an interesting property that derives from them.

The evolution shown in the first four graphs of Figure 4-9 agrees with what would be expected. The transition frequency and slew rate needed to comply with the given total settling time increase as the step amplitude increases. This makes the total consumption to increase and the optimum g_m/I_D ratios to decrease. The optimum pair of g_m/I_D ratios of the input and output stages features, as in the case of the example analyzed above, higher g_m/I_D at the output stage. This result is explained later. For higher step amplitudes the slew rate has, as expected, more influence, and thus the percentage of linear settling that leads to optimum consumption decreases with increasing step amplitude. The compensation capacitor of the optimum design decreases with increasing amplitude, which is reasonable since the transition frequency is rising.

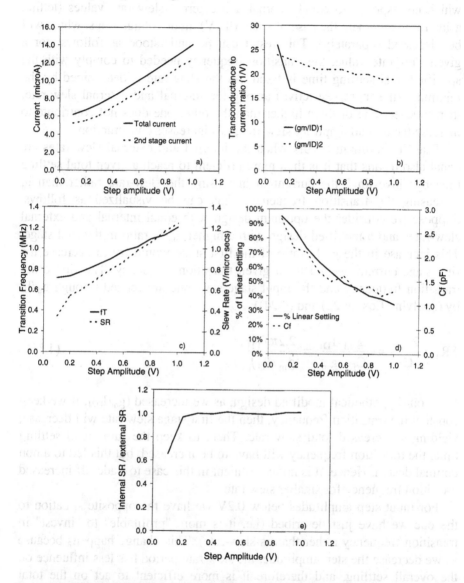

Figure 4-9. Evolution of characteristics of optimum design for total settling time of 1μs on a 10pF load as a function of the output step amplitude. a) Total current and second stage current, b) input ($(g_m/I_D)1$) and output ($(g_m/I_D)2$) stage transconductance to current ratio, c) first order transition frequency (f_T) and slew rate (SR), d) percentage of linear settling and compensation capacitance, e) ratio of internal to external slew rate.

A new, interesting result is found in Figure 4-9 e). The optimum is achieved for the ratio between the input stage g_m/I_D and output stage g_m/I_D which corresponds to equal internal and external slew rate values (letting aside for the moment the case of small (0.1V) input voltage steps, which will be discussed separately). This result can be understood as follows: for a given slew rate value, the transition frequency needed to comply with the specified total settling time is fixed. As the slew rate is determined by the minimum (the more restrictive) among the internal and external slew-rate, then to select one of them higher than the other one does not contribute to increase the overall amplifier slew-rate, just increases consumption.

That the optimum occurs when the internal and external slew rates are equal also means that it is then more efficient to reach a given total settling time by "investing" the current in increasing the slew-rate rather than in increasing the transition frequency. This can be visualized as follows. Suppose we consider the optimum design with equal internal and external slew-rates and a modified design with a higher g_m/I_D ratio in the first stage. This increase in the g_m/I_D ratio of the first stage would try to decrease the first stage current needed for a given transition frequency. The first order transition frequency and the input stage slew rate are related through g_m/I_D by (applying Eqs. (4.22) and (4.24)):

$$SR_1 = \frac{2 \cdot I_{D1}}{C_f} = \frac{2 \cdot g_{m1}}{C_f} \frac{I_{D1}}{g_{m1}} = \frac{2 \cdot 2\pi \cdot f_{T1}}{(g_m/I_D)_1} \qquad (4.31)$$

In our hypothetical modified design, as we increased $(g_m/I_D)_1$, if we keep constant the transition frequency, then the first stage slew rate will decrease, yielding a decreased total slew rate. Then, to keep the same total settling time, the transition frequency will have to be increased, but this led to a non optimal design. Hence, it is not convenient in this case to trade-off increased transition frequency for smaller slew rate.

For input step amplitudes below 0.2V we have the opposite situation to the one we have just described (i.e. it is more "profitable" to "invest" in transition frequency rather than is slew-rate). This change happens because as we decrease the step amplitude, the slew rate period has less influence on the overall settling, and therefore it is more efficient to act on the total settling time through the transition frequency. When this occurs, we gain more from increasing the input stage g_m/I_D ratio, through the effect that this has on reducing the input stage current for a given transition frequency, in spite that this transition frequency has to be slightly increased to compensate for the reduction in slew rate that this increase of g_m/I_D provokes. This change of "strategy" at 0.2V is also visible in Figure 4-9 c), where we can see that for amplitudes of less than 0.2V, the decrease of the f_T with decreasing amplitude slows down while the decrease of the slew rate is more acute.

The condition of equal internal and external slew rates implies that the g_m/I_D ratio of the output stage is higher than the one of the input stage. This can be shown as follows. The internal and external slew rates are given by:

$$SR_{int} = \frac{2.I_{D1}}{C_f} = \frac{2.I_{D1}}{g_{m1}}\frac{g_{m1}}{C_f} = \frac{2.w_T}{\left(g_m\middle/I_D\right)_1} \tag{4.32}$$

$$SR_{ext} = \frac{I_{D2}}{C_2} = \frac{I_{D2}}{g_{m2}}\frac{g_{m2}}{C_2} = \frac{w_{ndp}}{\left(\dfrac{C_f}{C_1 + C_f\left(\dfrac{C_1}{C_2}+1\right)}\right)}\frac{1}{\left(g_m\middle/I_D\right)_2} \tag{4.33}$$

Then to have equal SR_{int} and SR_{ext} implies:

$$\frac{2.w_T}{\left(g_m\middle/I_D\right)_1} = \frac{w_{ndp}}{\left(\dfrac{C_f}{C_1 + C_f\left(\dfrac{C_1}{C_2}+1\right)}\right)}\frac{1}{\left(g_m\middle/I_D\right)_2}$$

$$\Rightarrow \frac{\left(g_m\middle/I_D\right)_2}{\left(g_m\middle/I_D\right)_1} = \frac{1}{2}\frac{w_{ndp}}{w_T}\frac{1}{\left(\dfrac{C_f}{C_1 + C_f\left(\dfrac{C_1}{C_2}+1\right)}\right)} > \frac{1}{2}\frac{w_{ndp}}{w_T} \tag{4.34}$$

The term $(1/2)(w_{ndp}/w_T)$ is determined by the stability condition. In our case we took $w_{ndp} = 2.2w_T$ so this terms equals 1.1. The ratio of the second and first stage g_m/I_D values exceeds this value by a factor that depends on the parasitic capacitance C_1. In the example of Figure 4-9, $(g_m/I_D)_2$ ranges from 1.35 to 1.58 times $(g_m/I_D)_1$ for input step amplitudes between 0.2V and 1.0V.

The plots in Figure 4-10 a) to e) show the evolution of the optimum design with the specified total settling time for fixed step amplitude of 0.5V.

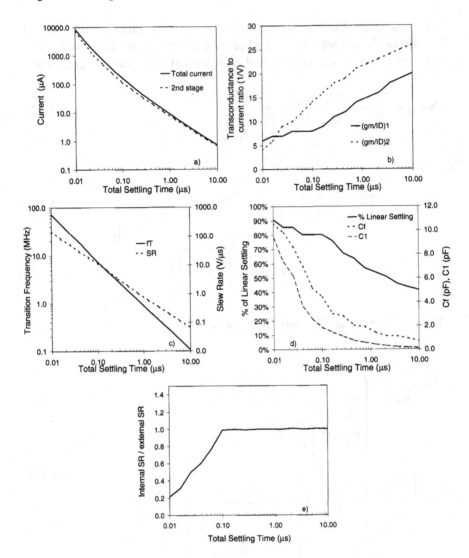

Figure 4-10. Evolution of characteristics of optimum design for a step amplitude of 0.5V on a 10pF load as a function of the total settling time. a) Total current and second stage current, b) input $((g_m/I_D)_1)$ and output $((g_m/I_D)_2)$ stage transconductance to current ratio, c) first order transition frequency (f_T) and slew rate (SR), d) percentage of linear settling, compensation capacitance and parasitic capacitance at the output of the first stage, e) ratio of internal to external slew rate.

The graphs a), b) c) follow the expected trends. As we decrease the specified total settling time, the consumption, transition frequency and slew rate increase, while the g_m/I_D ratios decrease. Graph d) shows that as we decrease the total settling time, the percentage of linear settling increases. Graph d) also shows a result that might seem surprising at first look: the required compensation capacitance increases as we decrease the total settling time. This happens although at the same time an increased transition frequency is needed. The explanation derives from the examination of the other curve that is plotted in graph d). This curve represents the parasitic capacitance at the output of the input stage (C_1), which is also increasing with decreasing total settling time, due to the increased transistor sizes required. Hence, an increased compensation capacitance is needed.

The plot e) shows the same behavior that was observed as a function of the step amplitude. For higher settling times, the optimum occurs when the internal and external slew rates are equal. As the specified settling time decreases, we get to a point (in this case at a settling time of about 100ns) where the percentage of time that the circuit is in linear settling is high enough, so that in order to further decrease the total settling time, it pays more to increase the transition frequency, in spite of a reduction of the slew-rate.

We will now discuss the influence of three parameters that have been considered fixed in the previous analysis: the load capacitance, the ratio of the non dominant pole frequency to the transition frequency (or equivalently the phase margin) and current mirror g_m/I_D ratio.

2.3.1 Effect of the load capacitance

The previous results have considered a 10pF load capacitance. We will now show that the characteristics of the optimum design (g_m/I_D values and internal to external slew rate ratio) remain the same independently of the load capacitance value. First, the studies of Figure 4-9 and Figure 4-10 were repeated for load capacitances of 3pF and 50pF. Then, the evolution of the optimum design as a function of the load capacitance for 0.5V step amplitude and 1µs total settling time was calculated. The following graphs present the results of these studies. Figure 4-11 a), b) and c) compare the evolution of the optimum design as a function of the step amplitude, for the three values of the load capacitance C_2 (3 pF, 10 pF and 50 pF). A total settling time of 1µs was considered in all cases. Figure 4-11 a) plots the g_m/I_D ratios of the input and output stages; in Figure 4-11 b) the ratio of internal to external slew rate is presented and Figure 4-11 c) shows the total consumption. From Figure 4-11 a) and b), it can be seen that the optimum combination of g_m/I_D ratios and the criterion of having equal internal and external slew rate remain valid when the load capacitance is changed. The small variations between the curves corresponding to different load capacitances are due to the discrete steps applied in the g_m/I_D ratios and C_f values in the exploration of the design space. For input step values (or total settling times values, as shown below) where the criterion of equal internal and external slew rate holds, other optimum values are equally unaffected by the change in the load capacitance. These are the optimum values of transition frequency, slew rate and time fraction in linear settling and in slew rate mode. The change in the load capacitance does affect other variables such as the compensation capacitance value and the currents, as is illustrated in Figure 4-11 c) for the case of the total consumption.

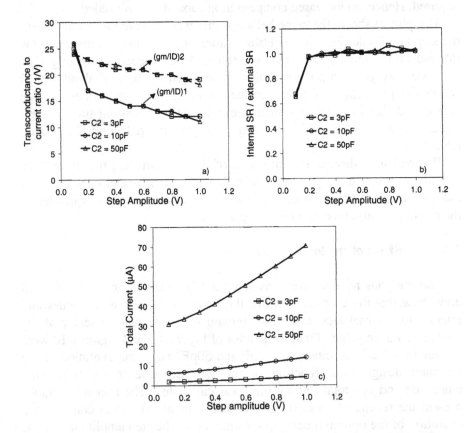

Figure 4-11. Effect of the value of the load capacitance on the characteristics of the optimum design when considered as a function of the step amplitude for a total settling time of 1μs. a) Input $((g_m/I_D)_1)$ and output $((g_m/I_D)_2)$ stage transconductance to current ratio, b) ratio of internal to external slew rate, c) total current. The results for 3pF, 10pF and 50pF loads are marked with square, circle and triangle symbols respectively.

The independence of the previous results from the value of the load capacitance is also supported by the results shown in Figure 4-12 and in Figure 4-13. The plots in Figure 4-12 a), b) and c) are analogous to those of Figure 4-11 when the variation with total settling time, for an amplitude step of 0.5V is considered. Figure 4-13 considers the evolution with the load capacitance of the optimum consumption for a design with a fixed step amplitude of 0.5V and total settling time of 1μs.

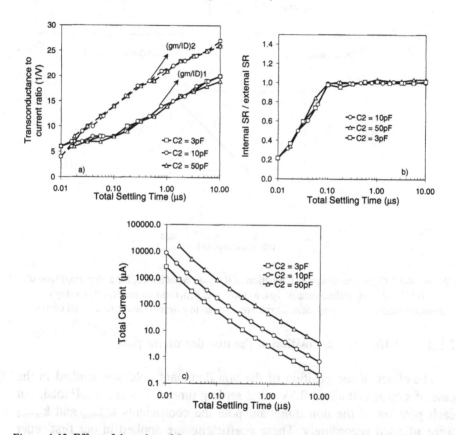

Figure 4-12. Effect of the value of the load capacitance on the characteristics of the optimum design when considered as a function of the total settling time when for a step amplitude of 0.5V. a) Input $((g_m/I_D)_1)$ and output $((g_m/I_D)_2)$ stage transconductance to current ratio, b) ratio of internal to external slew rate, c) total current. The results for 3pF, 10pF and 50pF loads are marked with square, circle and triangle symbols respectively.

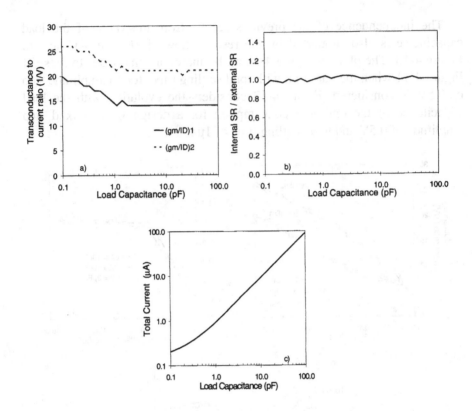

Figure 4-13. Optimum design as a function of the load capacitance, for a step amplitude of 0.5V and total settling time of 1μs. a) Input (($g_m/I_D)_1$) and output (($g_m/I_D)_2$) stage transconductance to current ratio, b) ratio of internal to external slew rate, c) total current.

2.3.2   Effect of the position of the non dominant pole

The effect of the position of the non dominant pole was studied in the case of step amplitude of 0.5V, total settling time of 1μs and 10pF load. For each position of the non dominant pole the coefficients $k_{corrsetl}$ and k_{corrwT} were adjusted accordingly. These coefficients are applied in our first order model in order to introduce the change in settling time due to the change in settling behavior ($k_{corrsetl}$) and time constant value (k_{corrwT}) due to a second order system. Figure 4-14 a) depicts the total current consumption and value of the correction coefficients as a function of the position of the non-dominant pole with respect to the transition frequency of the first order system. Figure 4-14 b) shows the evolution of the internal to external slew rate ratio with the position of the non dominant pole.

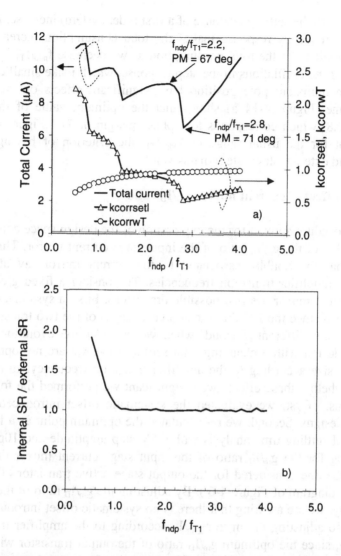

Figure 4-14. Effect of the position of the non dominant pole on the optimum performance. a) Total current consumption and correction coefficients $k_{corrsetl}$, k_{corrwT}, b) ratio of internal to external slew rate.

Let us analyze the behavior of the magnitudes plotted in Figure 4-14 a) as we decrease the ratio of the non dominant pole f_{ndp} to the gain-bandwidth product (here noted f_{T1} as the transition frequency of the equivalent first order system). On the one hand, the actual transition frequency decreases with respect to the transition frequency of the first order system, hence k_{corrwT} decreases. On the other hand the step response becomes more oscillatory, making the correction coefficient $k_{corrsetl}$ (which takes into account the difference with the settling response of a first order system) increase. A more oscillatory frequency response makes the total consumption increase. The non monotonicity of the total consumption as we decrease f_{ndp}/f_{T1} is due to the effect of the oscillations in the step response, which make small changes in the non dominant pole position have significant effects on the linear settling time. Figure 4-14 a) shows that the optimum value of the ratio f_{ndp}/f_{T1} is 2.8, which corresponds to a phase margin of 71°. Figure 4-14 b) shows that for the usual range of f_{ndp}/f_{T1}, the criterion of having equal internal and external slew-rate remains valid.

2.3.3   Effect of current mirror g_m/I_D ratio

The procedure applied for the exploration of the design space considered a fixed value of the g_m/I_D ratio of the input stage current mirror. This value assured that the doublet associated to the current mirror lay after the considered amplifier transition frequencies. To consider a fixed g_m/I_D ratio for the current mirror has two possible drawbacks. First, a systematic offset is introduced since the DC drain to source voltages of the two transistors of the mirror are different. Second, when we consider the evolution of the optimum design with a changing total settling time, we are not optimizing the mirror size according to the amplifier transition frequency. In order to quantify whether these effects were significant we performed the following calculations. First, we evaluated the systematic offset introduced in the previous designs. Second, we re-calculated the optimum point as a function of the total settling time analysis with 0.5V step amplitude and 10pF load, considering for the g_m/I_D ratio of the input stage current mirror the same value as the one considered for the output stage active transistor (T_2 in the schematic diagram of Figure 4-6). By adjusting the g_m/I_D ratio of the mirror in this way, we are assuring that there is no systematic offset introduced and we are also adjusting the mirror g_m/I_D according to the amplifier transition frequency, since the optimum g_m/I_D ratio of the output transistor will move towards strong inversion as the amplifier transition frequency increases.

The results of these calculations are as follows. In the original procedure, with a fixed current mirror g_m/I_D ratio, the systematic offset introduced varies from 0.5mV for a total settling time of 10µs to 2.6mV for a total settling time of 10ns. Therefore the systematic offset introduced would be, at most, only comparable with the random offset. The results for the optimum calculated with equal g_m/I_D ratios for the mirror and output transistors, as a function of the transition frequency were practically identical to the original results.

2.3.4 Comparison of optimum consumption in FD SOI and Bulk technologies

Finally, these results of optimum consumption in FD SOI technology were compared to those achievable in Bulk technology. The same procedure for the exploration of the design space was applied with the process data of a comparable Bulk technology, which was given in Chapter 3. To make a comparison in similar conditions, the g_m/I_D ratio of the input stage current mirror was chosen so that it provided the same current mirror pole frequency as the one we have in FD SOI technology. In FD SOI the current mirror pole frequency, calculated according the procedure presented in Chapter 3 is 89MHz for 3µm length and a g_m/I_D ratio of 10 V^{-1} in the current mirror. We must remember this is an estimation that does not consider additional parasitic capacitances connected to the current mirror input. To reach the same pole frequency in bulk, a g_m/I_D ratio of 5 V^{-1} is needed.

The ratio of total consumption of Bulk to SOI ranged from 1.18 to 1.66 for settling times in the 100µs down to 40ns range. It must pointed out that the bulk design will be worst in several aspects that are improved in SOI, such as gain, input common mode range and output voltage swing. If we would aim to equalize these aspects in both designs, the savings in consumption in SOI would rise. Figure 4-15 shows the optimum consumption and resulting g_m/I_D ratios in both technologies.

3. EVALUATION AND CONCLUSIONS

This chapter has discussed the factors that determine power consumption in analog circuits, proceeding from the theoretical limits to an example of methodology to optimize power consumption in the design of an operational amplifier.

In the first part the theoretical and practical limits to power consumption as well as the figures of merit of the power efficiency of analog circuits have been reviewed. One consequence of this analysis for the evaluation of the results of our sense channel case of study is that the minimum power consumption of a circuit that provides voltage gain is proportional to this gain. This conclusion is relevant when comparing the consumption of the filter/amplifier of the sense channel design with the consumption of filters that are usually designed for unity in-band gain.

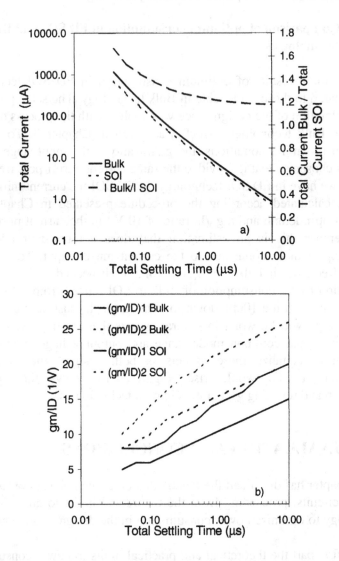

Figure 4-15. Optimum consumption (a) and g_m/I_D ratio (b) in Bulk and SOI as a function of the total settling time, for a 0.5V step amplitude and 10pF load capacitor. The g_m/I_D ratios of the current mirror transistors are 10 V^{-1} in SOI and 5 V^{-1} in Bulk.

The second part presents a systematic study on the partition of the total settling time between the slew rate dominated period and the linear settling period in order to optimize power consumption. Our study is based on a simple, design-oriented model for the total settling time, which, contrary to previous works, includes the modeling of both internal and external slew rates and considers a general feedback factor β. The proposed design procedure was tested in the case of a Miller RC compensated OTA but it can be easily generalized to other OTA architectures. The resulting exploration of the design space provides the optimum values of the g_m/I_D ratios for the input and output transistors as well as the optimum combination between slewing and linear settling periods. We have shown that an optimum exists and we have given a method to determine it. Moreover, the results show that this optimum complies, for ample ranges of input step amplitudes, with the property of being the design that leads to equal internal and external slew rate values.

The proposed method can be applied in a loop in order to adjust other performance aspects that are not considered in the optimization. For instance, DC gain, offset and 1/f noise can be improved if necessary by increasing the transistor lengths and repeating the procedure. In certain cases, it might be necessary to choose a solution that is "sub-optimal". This would be the case, for example, if the resulting input common mode range and output swing (which are related to the g_m/I_D ratios of the input and output stages) are not sufficient. Nevertheless, even in this case the method provide us with a very suitable starting point for further optimizations.

The proposed approach is an example of the superior properties of the g_m/I_D method proposed in [SIL96] as a tool to explore the design space.

Chapter 5

Class AB Micropower Operational Amplifiers

Class AB amplifiers contribute to minimize power in several ways: on the one hand by decoupling the large signal (i.e. slew rate and current through the load resistor), and small signal (i.e. stability) requirements on the output stage; on the other hand by reducing quiescent current consumption when the signal to be processed, as in this case the cardiac signal, is "active" during only a small part of the system cycle. When a class A amplifier is applied, as was the case of the pacemaker sense channel described in Chapter 2, the class A bias current, which is consumed permanently, must be dimensioned according to the output current demand when a large signal is applied. However, this large signal is only present during a very small part of the system cycle.

This chapter presents a novel approach for the design of a class AB output stage suitable for a micropower environment ([SIL00]).

Most work in the "mainstream" class AB design stems from either power amplifiers (e.g. audio power amplifiers); buffers and amplifiers for very low load impedance (e.g. line drivers); or "general purpose" op. amp. cells and "off-the-shelf" op. amp. design, which are specified for dealing with loads in the kΩ / hundreds of pF range. Some work has also been devoted to amplifiers for switched capacitor filters, which is an area closer to our goals.

Our central goal is to obtain a design suitable to replace the second stage in a two stage Miller amplifier for the sense channel application. Detailed specifications of this amplifier were presented in Chapters 1 and 2. These specifications call for characteristics that are not commonly addressed together in "mainstream" class AB architectures:
a) Micropower consumption
b) Operation at 2V power supply
c) Load with high resistance (some MΩs) and medium capacitance (50pF)

123

d) Need for well-controlled quiescent current, independent of supply
   voltage, which will vary in a large range.

Usual class AB designs, that aim at dealing with low load impedances,
end up with complex structures that induce big penalties in terms of base
quiescent current (due to many auxiliary circuits), area and design
complexity.

On the other hand some simple structures (e.g. the one shown in Fig. 4.70
of [GRE86] at page 181) have quiescent current which is greatly dependent
on the supply voltage.

Consequently, our general goal was to develop a *simple, low-voltage,
very low consumption* structure *aimed at replacing class A output stages* for
high load resistance / medium load capacitance amplifiers. Though the direct
application is the pacemaker sense channel, more general application
domains are active RC filters, MOSFET-C filters and switched capacitors
filters. The proposed method was experimentally tested for transition
frequencies up to more than 10MHz in 2 μm Fully-Depleted SOI and 0.8 μm
Bulk CMOS technologies.

This chapter will be organized as follows. First, we will introduce the
general characteristics of class AB stages and review the main structures
found in the literature. Then, we will describe the selected architecture and
the method applied to synthesize it for minimum power consumption.
Particular attention will be devoted in this part to the modeling of the high
frequency doublets introduced by the current mirrors. Next, the experimental
results on the fabricated prototypes and comparisons with reported
amplifiers of similar characteristics will be presented. Finally, improvements
to the basic circuit structure and design method will be discussed.

1.   GENERAL CHARACTERISTICS AND STRUCTURES OF CLASS AB STAGES

1.1   General characteristics

An output stage is based on two blocks: one that sources current from the
positive power supply to the load and another one that sinks current from the
load to ground or the negative power supply. In class A stages the signal is
delivered to the load only through one of these blocks, while the other one is
a constant bias current source (Figure 5-1 a)). In class AB and class B stages,
the signal reaches the load through both blocks (Figure 5-1 b)). The
difference between class AB and B lies in the current flowing through these
blocks when in quiescent conditions, i.e. when there is no current delivered

to the load. The quiescent current through the class B output devices is null, while in class AB there exists a minimum current in order to guarantee stability and improve the linearity of the stage at low amplitude output signals (i.e. avoid crossover distortion).

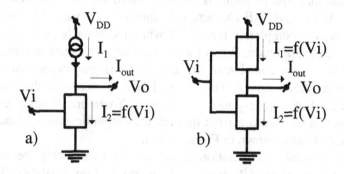

Figure 5-1. Basic structure of a) class A and b) class AB stages.

A standard way to graphically describe the current characteristics of an output stage [LAN99, SJO99] is with the plot of the stage source current (I_1 in Figure 5-1 b)) and sink current (I_2 in Figure 5-1 b)) as a function of the output current I_{out}. Current characteristics are shown in Figure 5-2 a) for a class A stage and in Figure 5-2 b) and c) for typical class AB stages. The characteristic of Figure 5-2 b) summarizes the main operating principles of class AB stages. At zero output current there is a non-zero current through the output devices I_Q. As the magnitude of I_{out} increases, one of the output devices delivers the load current while the other one tends to cut-off in order to increase the efficiency.

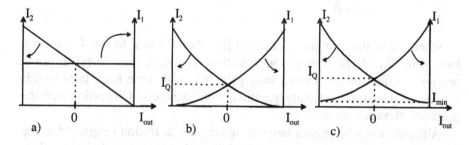

Figure 5-2. Plots of current characteristics of a) class A stage, b) class AB stage, c) class AB with minimum current I_{min}

The main specifications of a class AB output stage are determined as follows. The quiescent current must assure the stability (i.e. the desired small-signal phase margin) for a given load capacitance. The maximum current that the stage can deliver must be sufficient for supplying the current through the load resistor at maximum output amplitude and for supplying the required current through the load capacitor (i.e. for assuring the desired output or external slew rate).

An additional improvement is often imposed on the operation of class AB stages. In the class AB characteristic shown in Figure 5-2 b), one of the output devices is completely turned off when the other is supplying a load current of large amplitude. When the device that is off must conduct again, a delay appears, associated with the action of charging capacitances at the output device or its driver. This delay leads to increased distortion and ringing in the transient response of the stage. Therefore, it is preferable to always assure a minimum current through the output devices as done by the current characteristic shown in Figure 5-2 c).

A final general consideration refers to the relationship between the characteristics of class AB stages and distortion. Low distortion is not a critical feature in the pacemaker sense channel amplifier; nevertheless, the analysis of the distortion characteristics of the proposed class AB stages is important when considering their more general application. The main principle here is that for given open loop nonlinearities, the distortion in a closed loop configuration depends on the amount of loop gain at the frequency of interest [CAS92]. This principle is a consequence of the well-known property of feedback of reducing gain sensitivity and distortion [GRA93, pp.537, 538]. It can be exemplified as follows. Consider a two stage amplifier in which the output stage gain (A_2) is non linear, i.e. its gain is dependent on the output signal. The closed loop gain A_{cl} is given by:

$$A_{cl} = \frac{A_1.A_2}{1 + A_1.A_2.\beta} \tag{5.1}$$

where A_1 is the first stage gain and β is the feedback factor. If the open loop gain $(A_1. A_2.\beta)$ is much greater than 1, the A_2 non linearity has a negligible effect on the closed loop gain. We will come back later to this expression in order to estimate quantitatively the expected distortion with the proposed class AB stage.

Although open loop gain helps to reduce the distortion originated at the output stage, to lower the root causes of distortion is always desirable. This means a flat stage gain with small variation with I_{out}, for both positive and negative values of I_{out}. This is an objective pursued in many class AB architectures [LAN99]. Nevertheless, we will show that due to the reduction achieved through the loop gain, architectures that deliberately have non-symmetrical gain for positive and negative I_{out}, still achieve very reasonable distortion values (-60dB).

1.2 Structures

Traditional class AB stages applied the common drain configuration (or common collector in bipolar technology) for the output devices. This is not acceptable in a low supply voltage environment, since the output swing is reduced by one gate-source or base-emitter voltage at each supply rail. Low voltage stages apply common source output devices as shown in Figure 5-3. Consequently, the stage is capable of providing voltage gain, which is a feature we need since we will apply the class AB stage to replace a class A stage in a two stage amplifier.

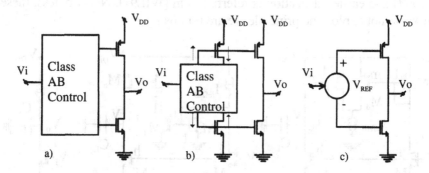

Figure 5-3. a) General common source class AB stage, b) Feedback class AB control, c) Feedforward class AB control.

Once we have defined the configuration of the output devices we need a mechanism to drive the gate of the output transistors from the input signal so that we have a class AB current characteristic as shown in Figure 5-2 b) or c) and a well controlled quiescent current. This class AB control is done in two ways in existing stages [LAN99]: feedback control and feedforward control.

In feedback control (Figure 5-3 b)) the current through the output devices is sensed and then the class AB control acts in a feedback loop on the output transistor gates, in order to achieve a given class AB operation and quiescent current. In feedforward control there is no feedback; the voltage driving the gates is generated directly from the input, relying only on matching to set the output transistors class AB operation. A way of implementing the feedforward strategy is to simulate a floating voltage source that controls the output transistor gates as in Figure 5-3 c). Feedback strategies allow to design and control the class AB characteristic more precisely, although they have the added difficulty of dealing with a feedback loop that must be kept stable, within an already complex op-amp scheme.

An ample review on these two alternatives with several examples of implementations is found in [LAN99] as well as in [CAS92].

2.   PROPOSED CLASS AB ARCHITECTURE

The structures we applied here are shown in Figure 5-4.a and Figure 5-4.b [SIL00]. The quiescent current is determined through a feedback loop that senses the current through M_a (with transistor M_f) and adjusts the quiescent current, acting on the current through the output transistor M_b. The structure of Figure 5-4.b has been applied previously in [VER96] and [GRI97] and earlier utilization is referred to in [WIL91]. Nevertheless, these works do not exploit the principle we are proposing.

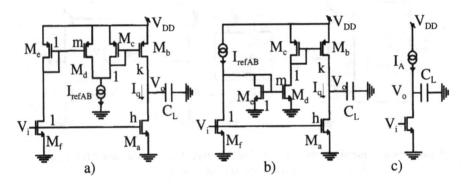

Figure 5-4. Class AB output stages (a, b) and conventional class A output stage (c). From [SIL021], © 2002 IEEE.

The design approach we propose provides a significant reduction in power consumption with respect to traditional class AB and class A structures by three means. First, the output stage transconductance is boosted through the current mirror gains resulting in an important improvement of its transconductance to current ratio. Second, it can be shown that this increase in the output stage transconductance, results in a reduction of the value of the Miller compensation capacitor that gives minimum consumption for a complete amplifier. This reduction in the compensation capacitor, besides saving area, makes it possible to reduce the first stage consumption and to operate the first stage transistor closer to weak inversion. This provides additional benefits in terms of increased input common mode range and reduced offset voltage. Third, the architecture provides a low impedance path from the input of the driver stage to the output transistors, avoiding compensating capacitors internal to the output stage.

Besides the improvement in power consumption, the circuit is also very well suited for low-voltage operation. The output stage only requires one gate –source plus one source –drain voltage to operate. In addition, these voltages are reduced due to the lower current required thanks to the transconductance multiplication effect.

Two disadvantages appear with respect to more complex class AB architectures.

First, no mechanism is provided to assure that both output branches will always remain in conduction. This, as mentioned above, leads to increased ringing in the time response for high amplitude steps and increased distortion, due to the increased turn-on delay associated to the branch that is cut off. This disadvantage is of no consequence in the case of the pacemaker sense channel application, due to the kind of signals that are handled, though it could be of concern in other applications. Moreover, this point can be solved with a simple addition to the stage structure, implying small penalties on consumption and minimum supply voltage as described later.

Second, the ratio of the maximum output current to the quiescent current is fixed by the current mirror gains. As we will see below, the maximum allowable value of these gains is limited due to its effect on stability. Thus, the ratio of maximum output current to quiescent current is also limited. In spite of the last disadvantage, a significant reduction in consumption with respect to a class A case is achieved.

Distortion is an additional possible concern, when considering the use of this architecture in general applications, besides the pacemaker case. The transconductance multiplication effect is based on an asymmetric behavior of the p and n sections of the output stage, hence leading to a non linear behavior of the output stage. However, as we discussed above and we will demonstrate based on estimations and measurements shown below, the high gain allows us to reach very reasonable distortion figures.

Concerning the comparison of the architectures of Figure 5-4 a) and b), the b) architecture is more efficient; for a given quiescent current I_q in the output branch and equal gains of the current mirrors, the total consumption is higher for architecture a). For usual values of gains of the current mirrors shown below, the total current increase for architecture a) can be in the range of 1 to 3 times I_q.

On the other hand, architecture a) is more apt for high frequency operation for the reasons that follow. In architecture b) one aspect limiting the high frequency operation is the frequency response of current mirror M_e – M_d . This mirror has a small current through M_e, since its current is the output branch quiescent current divided by the product k times m. We are interested in increasing this product, since this will increase the transconductance multiplication effect. In addition, in architecture b), the parasitic capacitance that fixes the pole of the mirror $M_e - M_d$ is increased by the parasitic capacitance of the current source I_{refAB}.

In the architecture a) the current through M_e is higher (which makes this stage to be less efficient). On the other hand, M_e-M_d are in the a) case pMOS transistors instead of nMOS, but this is usually compensated by the increase in current. If this stage would be used with a first stage with an nMOS differential pair, the symmetric stages, interchanging p-type and n-type transistor, would be used and the architecture a) would have a further advantage in frequency response.

Since we are looking for solutions that favor consumption reduction, in what follows we will consider architecture b).

We will now analyze the main characteristics of the proposed approach.

The quiescent current is fixed with respect to the I_{refAB} current source as follows. In quiescent conditions, the output current at the V_o terminal is zero and the output branch quiescent current (I_q in Figure 5-4) must be such that the sum of the scaled versions of I_q at M_e and M_f is equal to I_{refAB}. This condition yields:

$$I_q = \frac{k.mI_{refAB}}{1 + \dfrac{k.m}{h}} \tag{5.2}$$

where h, k and m are the gain factors of the current mirrors shown in Figure 5-4

The total equivalent transconductance of this stage under class AB operation, defined as the ratio between the total signal output current i_o and the input signal voltage v_i is given by:

$$g_m = g_{ma}(1 + \frac{km}{h})D(s) \tag{5.3}$$

where g_{ma} is the transconductance of the output transistor M_a and $D(s)$ represents the contribution of the frequency response of the current mirrors. Although these may introduce high frequency doublets, the circuit can be properly stabilized even if the stage transconductance is multiplied by factors as high as 25.

It is also interesting to consider the effect on the transconductance to consumed current ratio (g_m/I_D) of the stage. It is given by:

$$(g_m / I_D) = (g_m / I_D)_a \cdot \frac{(1 + \dfrac{km}{h})}{(1 + \dfrac{1}{k} + \dfrac{1}{km} + \dfrac{1}{h})} D(s) \qquad (5.4)$$

In this case, multiplication factors as high as 12 can be achieved. This is like having an equivalent transistor 12 times more efficient than the original one.

Let us now consider the influence of the response of the current mirrors. The $D(s)$ factor is given by Eq. (5.5). The factor $(1+km/h)$ that multiplies the transconductance in Eq. (5.3) is noted by g_{mmult}, while w_c (resp. w_e) is the angular frequency of the pole of the current mirror M_b-M_c (resp. M_d-M_e). The latter is given by the ratio of the M_c (M_e) transconductance over the total capacitance at the M_c (M_e) gate node.

$$D(s) = \frac{1 + \left(\dfrac{1}{w_e} + \dfrac{1}{w_c}\right) \dfrac{s}{g_{mmult}} + \dfrac{1}{w_e w_c} \dfrac{s^2}{g_{mmult}}}{\left(1 + \dfrac{s}{w_e}\right)\left(1 + \dfrac{s}{w_c}\right)} \qquad (5.5)$$

The doublet introduces an important phase shift near the w_c and w_e frequencies. This phase shift increases with g_{mmult}, as shown in Figure 5-5. This effect determines the maximum acceptable values for the g_{mmult} factor. The next section shows the method applied to determine the optimum solution.

Let us now summarize the factors that determine the achievable total consumption reduction. Consider we apply this output stage as the second stage of a Miller amplifier, in which the Miller capacitance is connected between the V_i and V_o terminals of Figure 5-4.b. Since the non-dominant pole of this amplifier is proportional to the second stage transconductance, the second stage current will decrease in a proportion comparable to the increase in the g_m/I_D ratio, when compared to the class A output stage (shown in Figure 5-4.c). The improvement in g_m/I_D is not completely translated into a reduction of the current. The reason is that the non-dominant pole must be slightly increased, with respect to the class A case, to have the same phase margin while allowing the phase shift introduced by the doublets. Taking these factors into account, reductions of quiescent current by a factor of 3 to 4 with respect to the class A case are achievable.

Finally, we consider the maximum output current capability of the stage. The maximum source current is given by $k.m.I_{refAB}$, while the maximum sink current is limited by the size of M_a and the maximum V_i voltage at the input of the stage.

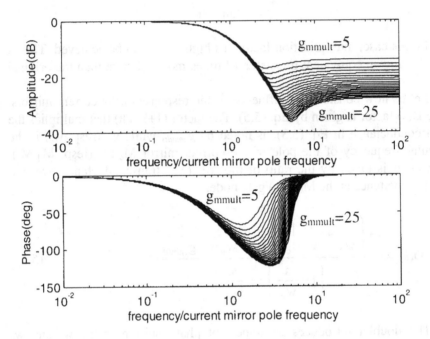

Figure 5-5. Amplitude and phase of the current mirrors frequency response D(s) for both current mirror poles located at the same frequency. The response is shown as a function of the frequency normalized to the current mirror pole frequency. The transconductance multiplication factor g_{mmult} varies from 5 to 25.

3.   DESIGN METHOD

A design methodology for the application of this output stage to a Miller amplifier with R-C compensation network was developed. The R-C network eliminates the right half plane zero of the Miller amplifier making it possible to reduce the overall consumption by further decreasing the requirements on the second stage transconductance. The input stage uses a simple pMOS differential pair. The amplifier schematic is shown in Figure 5-6.

The phase margin of this amplifier is determined by the position of the non dominant pole with respect to the transition frequency and by the response of the current mirrors. This last factor, as shown in Eq. (5.5), depends only on the frequency of the poles and the gain of the mirrors (through g_{mmult}). Let us express this relationship by the following equation:

$$PM = f\left({}^{w_{ndp0}}\!\!\diagup\!\!_{w_T}, w_c, w_e, k, h, m \right) \tag{5.6}$$

where w_{ndp0} is the Miller amplifier non dominant pole angular frequency that would result if the influence of the frequency response of the current mirrors were negligible, (i.e. $D(s) = 1$):

$$w_{ndp0} = \frac{g_{ma}\left(1 + \dfrac{k.m}{h}\right)}{\dfrac{C_1 C_2}{C_f} + C_2 + C_1} \tag{5.7}$$

where C_f is the Miller compensating capacitance, C_1 is the parasitic capacitance at the input of the output stage and C_2 is the load capacitance.

Later we will discuss the exact expression to be applied as Eq. (5.6)

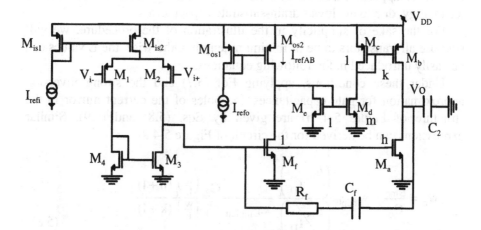

Figure 5-6. Complete Miller RC compensated OTA with class AB output stage. From [SIL00], © 2000 IEEE.

3.1   Selection of the gains of current mirrors

Since the gains of the current mirrors k, h and m, affect the amplifier phase margin (through their influence on the output stage transconductance and on the frequency response of the current mirrors) as well as the total quiescent current of the second stage, this trade-off between power and stability must be taken into account to design this amplifier.

We developed a design procedure based on finding the set of current mirror gains that provides the maximum reduction in consumption while preserving stability.

First, we derived simplified approximate analytical expressions for the current mirrors poles. The main goal was to allow to decouple different steps of the synthesis procedure like the selection of k, h and m, the sizing of the first stage transistors and the determination of the Miller capacitance that otherwise should be carried out through a more complex iterative process. These expressions are based on the following assumptions:

a) the parasitic capacitance at the input of the second stage C_1 is approximately given by the gate capacitance of M_a and M_f. It is supposed to be negligible with respect to the Miller capacitance C_f.

b) the gate capacitances also dominate in the parasitic capacitances that define the poles of the current mirrors (reasonable hypothesis when the current mirror factor is larger than 1).

These assumptions are valid in the amplifiers under consideration and are even more appropriate in the case of SOI technology than in Bulk CMOS technology, due to the lower drain-substrate capacitances.

For the sake of simplicity in the illustration of the procedure, we will suppose all transistors to be of minimum length. Otherwise, the L values can be easily introduced in the following equations.

Under these conditions, applying Eq. (5.7) and the strong inversion approximation for gate capacitances, the poles of the current mirror in the structure of Figure 5-4 b) are given by Eqs. (5.8) and (5.9). Similar expressions can be derived for the circuit of Figure 5-4 a).

$$w_c = \frac{g_{mc}}{C_c} \cong w_{ndp0} \cdot \frac{\left(g_m / I_D\right)_c}{\left(g_m / I_D\right)_a} \frac{1}{k \cdot g_{mmult}} \frac{C_2}{C_1} \frac{\left(\frac{W}{L}\right)_f (h+1)}{\left(\frac{W}{L}\right)_c (k+1)}$$

$$\cong w_{ndp0} \cdot \frac{1}{k \cdot g_{mmult}} \frac{C_2}{C_1} \frac{\left(\frac{W}{L}\right)_f (h+1)}{\left(\frac{W}{L}\right)_c (k+1)}$$

(5.8)

$$w_e = \frac{g_{me}}{C_e} \cong w_{ndp0} \cdot \frac{\left(g_m\big/I_D\right)_e}{\left(g_m\big/I_D\right)_a} \frac{1}{k.m.g_{mmult}} \frac{C_2}{C_1} \frac{\left(\frac{W}{L}\right)_f (h+1)}{\left(\frac{W}{L}\right)_e (m+1)}$$

(5.9)

$$\cong w_{ndp0} \frac{1}{k.m.g_{mmult}} \frac{C_2}{C_1} \frac{\left(\frac{W}{L}\right)_f (h+1)}{\left(\frac{W}{L}\right)_e (m+1)}$$

where $(g_m/I_D)_i$ is the transconductance over current ratio for transistor i (with i = a, e, c), and g_{mc} and C_c (g_{me} and C_e) are the transconductance and parasitic capacitance at the gate of transistor M_c (M_e).

In the third approximate expression in Eqs. (5.8) and (5.9), it was considered that the g_m/I_D values of transistors M_a, M_c and M_e which are in similar biasing conditions are approximately equal. A more exact procedure would be to express the quotients between g_m/I_D and (W/L) that appear in Eqs. (5.8) and (5.9) as a function of the g_m/I_D values and current ratios (i.e. current mirror gains). For the case of Eq. (5.8) this can be done as follows (and in analogous way for Eq. (5.9)):

$$\frac{\left(g_m\big/I_D\right)_c \big/ \left(\frac{W}{L}\right)_c}{\left(g_m\big/I_D\right)_a \big/ \left(\frac{W}{L}\right)_f} = \frac{\left(g_m\big/I_D\right)_c \big/ \left(\frac{W}{L}\right)_c}{\left(g_m\big/I_D\right)_a \big/ \left(\left(\frac{W}{L}\right)_a/h\right)} = \frac{\left(g_m\big/I_D\right)_c \left(I_{Dc}\big/\left(\frac{W}{L}\right)_c\right)}{\left(g_m\big/I_D\right)_a \left(I_{Da}\big/\left(\frac{W}{L}\right)_a\right)} \frac{I_{Da}}{I_{Dc}} \frac{1}{h}$$

$$= \frac{f\left(\left(g_m\big/I_D\right)_c\right)}{f\left(\left(g_m\big/I_D\right)_a\right)} \cdot \frac{k}{h}$$

(5.10)

where the last equality is obtained by applying an expression for the relationship of g_m/I_D vs. $I_D/(W/L)$ obtained from a transistor model continuous in all regions of operation, as was done in Chapter 3 to analyze the frequency response of the current mirror.

In any of these two approaches, the (g_m/I_D) or the (W/L) values that appear in Eqs. (5.8) and (5.9) are chosen a priori by the designer based on considerations such as transition frequency, output current and allowable bias voltages of internal nodes. Therefrom, considering equations (5.6), (5.8) and (5.9) we have a set of equations with the unknowns k, h, m and w_{ndp0}/w_T.

We then find, with the aid of an optimization program, the set of values which results in a given phase margin value while maximizing the ratio I_A/I_{AB} where I_A is the consumption of a class A output stage with the same phase margin and I_{AB} is the total quiescent current consumption of the class AB output stage.

We will now consider the issue of the calculation of the phase margin. The main contribution to the phase margin is through the term related to the non dominant pole in the amplifier open loop transfer function. Other contributions come from the input stage doublet [LAK94, pp. 622-627], and the zero and pole associated to the Miller resistor. The input stage doublet can be treated separately in the standard way and the pole and zero associated to the Miller resistor will be supposed to have a negligible influence, which is usually the case. The phase contributed by the non dominant pole is given by:

$$\text{phase}\left(\frac{1}{1+\dfrac{j.w}{w_{ndp0}.D(jw)}}\right)_{w=w_T} \tag{5.11}$$

where the dependence of the output stage transconductance g_{mo} (given by Eq. (5.3)) on the frequency response of the current mirrors $D(s)$, has been shown explicitly by expressing w_{ndp} as the product of w_{ndp0} (the non dominant pole angular frequency if the frequency response of the current mirrors were negligible) and the term $D(jw)$. Since the complex quantity $D(jw)$ influences the phase to be determined, the exact determination of this phase requires a numerical evaluation of Eq. (5.11). We initially took a simplified approach, which provides an approximate, pessimistic, estimation of the influence of the frequency response of the current mirrors on the phase margin. This simplified approach is to approximate the phase of Eq. (5.11) by:

$$\text{phase}\left(\frac{1}{1+\dfrac{j.w_T}{w_{ndp0}}}\right)+\text{phase}(D(j.w_T))=-a\tan\left(\frac{w_T}{w_{ndp0}}\right)+\text{phase}(D(j.w_T))$$

$$\tag{5.12}$$

where the second term is the one illustrated in Figure 5-5.

This second approach was the one applied in the design of the experimental prototypes presented in section 4. As shown there the achieved phase margin is indeed larger than the target goal of 60 degrees, which allows us to further increase the transition frequency. Alternatively, in section 5, where we discuss improvements to the design method and architecture, we present examples of calculated results when applying the exact phase margin given by Eq. (5.11) for the design.

3.2 Complete amplifier design

The complete amplifier design procedure can be summarized as follows:
1. First the (W/L) or g_m/I_D value for transistors M_c, M_e, and M_f is selected and the gain of the current mirrors k, h, m as well as the position of the non dominant pole w_{ndpo}/w_T are determined with the procedure described in section 3.1.
2. The lengths and g_m/I_D ratios of the transistors of the input stage transistors and bias current sources are selected.
3. We search for the C_f value that minimizes consumption for the required transition frequency and non dominant pole frequency, applying the g_m/I_D method [SIL96] for transistor sizing.
4. We verify whether the bias current of the output stage transistor M_a, I_{Da}, is enough to be able to source the maximum current demanded by the load.
This maximum load current is given by:

$$I_{L\max} = \frac{V_{op}}{R_2} + V_{op}.2.\pi.f_T.C_2 \tag{5.13}$$

where V_{op} is the peak output voltage and R_2 is the load resistance. Then it is verified whether:

$$I_{L\max} < I_{source\max} = I_{refAB}.k.m = I_{Da}.\left(\frac{1}{h} + \frac{1}{km}\right)km \tag{5.14}$$

If this relation does not hold for the I_{Da} determined according to the non dominant pole frequency, the minimum I_{Da} value that verifies this relation is selected.
5. If I_{Da} was changed in step 4 to comply with the load current requirements, then the output stage transistors are sized again according to the new I_{Da} value.
Some comments about this general design procedure arc due here.

a) This design procedure is not optimum in the sense that was proposed in Chapter 4, since it does not take jointly into account the internal and external slew rates. This procedure will usually lead to an amplifier whose slew rate is limited by the first stage to a much larger extent than the limit imposed by the output stage. Therefore, the design can be further optimized by not "oversizing" the output stage current. We took care of this aspect in the case of the amplifier for the pacemaker amplifier. In the other prototype amplifiers, that were planned as general purpose cells, since we were mostly interested in testing the output stage, we wanted it to be capable of handling different load configurations and therefore we preferred not to be "tight" on the current drive capability.

b) In step 4) the maximum load current is calculated based on requiring the stage to be capable of delivering a V_{op} output amplitude at a maximum frequency of f_T. This considers a worst case condition where the amplifier is applied in a follower configuration and we want to deliver an output signal without distortion up to the closed loop $-3dB$ frequency, which is equal to the amplifier f_T. In the case of the pacemaker amplifier we adapted this condition to the application by taking as maximum frequency the $-3dB$ frequency of the filter, which is 200 Hz.

3.3   Experimental prototypes

We successfully tested our approach to the design of the class AB output stage in the following experimental prototypes for 2V operation.

In 2µm FD SOI Technology:

A1: OTA for pacemaker sense channel

A2: OTA for 1MHz transition frequency

A3: OTA for 5 to 10MHz transition frequency

In 0.8µm Bulk Technology

A4: OTA for 14MHz transition frequency

A5 and A6: OTAs for switched capacitor implementation of the pacemaker sense channel.

Next, we summarize the resulting design data for amplifiers A1 to A4. Experimental measurement results are presented in the next section. Amplifiers A5 and A6 are described in the next chapter together with the switched capacitor implementation of the sense channel.

Table 5-1. Main design data of prototype class AB amplifiers.

	A1	A2	A3	A4
Target f_T (MHz)	0.16 (Note 1)	0.95	5.7	13.8
Load Cap. C_2 (pF)	50	20	5	5
Load Res. R_2 (kΩ)	6900	10	10	10
Total consumption (μA)	0.083	23	99	99
k	7	8	2	3
h	2	1	2	2
m	3	3	6	7
g_{mmult}	11.5	25	6	11.5
$(g_m/I_D)_{mult}$	6.8	11.5	2.9	6.1
C_f (pF)	0.25	1.35	1	0.2
R_f (Ω)	126,000	418	325	172
I_{refi} (μA)	0.01	0.5	1	1
I_{refo} (μA)	Note 2	0.5	2	5
Max. source current (μA)	0.315	247	312	557
Die area (mm^2)	0.030	0.063	0.060	0.010
Minimum transistor length used (μm)	3	3	2	0.8
Technology	FD SOI	FD SOI	FD SOI	Bulk

Note 1.: First order extrapolated f_T. The actual f_T is smaller, since the amplifier is not designed to be stable in unity gain configuration, it has the non dominant pole at 20kHz.

Note 2.: in this amplifier there is only one reference current; the output reference current is internally derived from the input reference current.

Analysis of the design results

It can be seen in Table 5-2 that the proposed method and architecture, through the increase of the second stage transconductance and reduction of the compensation capacitance, allows us to apply very high g_m/I_D ratios, particularly for the input transistors. This is even the case for amplifiers A3 and A4 which are aimed at transition frequencies of several MHz. Amplifier A1 takes advantage of g_m/I_D values (33 and 34 V^{-1}) close to the maximum provided by the technology. These high g_m/I_D ratios are applied jointly with extremely low bias currents (a few nA).

Amplifiers A3 and A4 have the same consumption while the transition frequency of amplifier A4 is much higher. This difference is misleading since it does not present a fair comparison between both amplifiers. The data of A3 in Table 5-1 are those coming from the synthesis procedure previously described, which applies Eq. (5.12) to estimate the phase margin and leads to a conservative design with a calculated phase margin of 80°. On the contrary the data for amplifier A4 derive from further modifying the initial design to increase the transition frequency. The transition frequency of A3 can be increased much closer to that of A4, while keeping an acceptable phase margin, as shown below in the experimental data.

Table 5-2. Transistor sizes, g_m/I_D ratios and quiescent bias currents for prototypes A1 to A4

	A1			A2			A3			A4		
	W /L (µm)	g_m/I_D (1/V)	I_D (nA)	W /L (µm)	g_m/I_D (1/V)	I_D (µA)	W /L (µm)	g_m/I_D (1/V)	I_D (µA)	W /L (µm)	g_m/I_D (1/V)	I_D (µA)
$M_{1,2}$	41 /9	33	8.3	280 /3	31	0.75	126 /2	25	1.5	24.5 /0.8	24	0.8
$M_{3,4}$	3.5 /24	24	8.3	48 /24	20	0.3	10 /2	17	1.5	2.8 /0.8	17	0.8
M_a	2 x 3 /3	30	27.4	30 /3	11	9.9	2 x 62 /2	13	44.6	48 /0.8	11	48.8
M_b	7 x 3 /3	30	27.4	8 x 3 /3	5	9.9	2 x 62 /2	8	44.6	72 /0.8	10	48.8
M_c	3 /3	30	3.9	3 /3	5	1.2	62 /2	8	22.3	24 /0.8	10	16.3
M_d	3 x 3 /3	34	3.9	3 x 3 /3	14	1.2	6 x 3 /2	7	22.3	14 /2	9	16.3
M_e	3 /3	34	1.3	3 /3	14	0.4	62 /2	7	3.7	2 /2	9	5.4
M_f	3 /3	30	13.7	30 /3	11	9.9	62 /2	13	22.3	24 / 0.8	11	24.4
M_{is1}	3.5 /6	25	10	37 /6	18	0.5	73.5 /6	18	1	3.2 / 2.4	9	1.0
M_{is2}	5.5 / 6	25	16.6	44.5 / 6	18	0.6	3 x 73.5 / 6	18	3	5.9 / 2.4	9	1.6
M_{os1}	Note 1	-	-	3 / 6	6	0.5	5 / 6	4	2	7 / 2.4	6	5.0
M_{os2}	5 / 6	25	15	52 / 6	6	10.3	59 / 6	4	26	5.3 x 7 / 2.4	6	26.5

Note 1.: Amplifier A1 does not use separate current mirrors for the input and output stages.

In addition, in order to compare amplifiers A3 and A4 on a common basis, we performed a synthesis starting from the specifications of amplifier A4 but for a 2µm bulk technology, comparable with the 2µm FD SOI technology of amplifier A3. As the determination of the k, h, and m gain factors does not consider the drain and source parasitic capacitances, only the gate capacitances, the result in this 2µm Bulk technology is the same as the result in the SOI technology (k=2, h=2, m=6). However, once these values are introduced into the amplifier design procedure, in order to be able to stabilize the bulk circuit, the m gain factor must be reduced from 6 to 5, reducing the g_{mmult} transconductance multiplication factor from 7 to 6. With this design the resulting total consumption is 245µA, and the calculated transition frequency and phase margin are 10.5MHz and 58°. This large increase in current consumption is explained by the decrease of the transconductance multiplication effect. The g_{mmult} factor was 11.5 in the 0.8µm bulk technology while only reaches 6 in the 2 µm bulk process. The increased parasitic capacitances in bulk with respect to SOI makes that the phase margin achievable in 2 µm bulk is much smaller than in 2 µm SOI, while the consumption increases from 99µA to 245µA.

The comparison of the A3 and A4 amplifiers and the impact of the difference of the minimal channel length in the bulk and SOI processes used will be further discussed hereunder, when the experimental data is presented.

Statistical simulation

Table 5-1 presents design data based on nominal process parameters. We now consider the effect of the fabrication spreads. This is done in the case of the 0.8 µm Bulk industrial process, where statistical data, provided by the foundry, are available. The results of a Monte Carlo simulation with 100 runs of amplifier A4 are shown in Table 5-3. The simulation conditions are 2V power supply, 0.7µA input stage bias current I_{refi}, 5µA output stage bias current I_{refo}, 5pF load capacitance and 100kΩ load resistor.

Table 5-3. Results of statistical simulation of amplifier A4.

	Nominal value	Standard deviation
Transition frequency (MHz)	13.2	1.4
Phase margin (°)	71	4.2
Quiescent supply current (µA)	95	14

It must be taken into account that these results are pessimistic as explained hereunder. In this simulation, some of the model parameters are randomly varied for each transistor. The tolerances applied might be representative for a random couple of transistors in the circuit, but they are not in the case of transistors with a layout intended to preserve their matching. This is verified in a Monte Carlo simulation of the output stage current mirrors $M_f - M_a$ and $M_c - M_b$, which use minimum length transistors. When these mirrors are simulated with the same bias current as in the final design and equal source to drain voltage at both sides of the mirror (i.e. letting aside the systematic error due to the finite output impedance), the standard deviation of the relative current error ranges from 7.7% for mirror $M_c - M_b$ to 32% for mirror $M_a - M_f$. These errors are too high, even for minimum length transistors, if the layout complies with basic matching rules. The pessimistic nature of these simulations is also shown by the results of the application of the Pelgrom matching model with typical matching parameters.

The spreads in transition frequency and phase margin achieved are, nevertheless, acceptable for most applications. Moreover, in spite of the pessimistic predictions of current mirror matching, which lead to a high spread in the quiescent current, the correct operation of the amplifier and its class AB output stage are maintained.

Die Area in SOI and Bulk

The similar characteristics of experimental prototypes of amplifier A3 and A4 allow us to consider them in order to compare SOI and Bulk technologies regarding the resulting die area. Table 5-4 provides data for this comparison. In the case of amplifier A3, the first row of Table 5-4 provides the actual die area as well as the die area scaled by the ratio of the square of the feature sizes of the processes applied in A4 and A3 (i.e. by $(0.8/2)^2$). Two die areas of amplifier A4 are provided, the first one is the die area of the fabricated amplifier, the second one, under the column "compact layout" refers to the die area resulting from a different floorplan, which leads to a more compact layout. From these data, we can conclude that both technologies lead to comparable die areas. As can be seen from Table 5-2, higher W/L ratios are sometimes applied in SOI, particularly in transistors operating in moderate and weak inversion. However, this increase in the gate area of transistors is approximately compensated by the higher area overhead of Bulk, due to the well used to implement complementary transistors on a common substrate and the need for contacts to the substrate or well. These compensating effects are evidenced in the data of the second and third rows of Table 5-4. The second row shows the sum of the gate area of the transistors (sum of the W.L products). The third row presents an indicator intended to compare the area overhead in both technologies. To evaluate this overhead the total area minus the area occupied by the compensation capacitor and resistor (C_f and R_f) is compared to the total transistor gate area. The results show that as discussed above, the approximately equal total die areas in Bulk and SOI for same process node, stem from the balance between a lower area overhead and a higher transistor gate area in SOI with respect to Bulk.

Table 5-4. Die area data for amplifiers A3 and A4.

	A3 Fabricated	A3 Scaled by $(0.8/2)^2$	A4 Fabricated	A4 Compact Layout
Die Area (μm^2)	60000	9600	10132	7980
Transistor Gate Area (Σ WL, μm^2)	3596	575	338	338
(Die area $- C_f$, R_f area) / Transistor Gate Area	14.5	14.5	29.6	23

Perspectives for scaled technologies

In order to assess the perspectives of the proposed architecture with scaling, the following estimation was done. We started from design A3 and synthesized it again with the process data of a 0.25µm FD SOI process [RAY98]. We kept the same length as in the original design for all transistors, in order to preserve the gain, except for transistors M_e and M_d which were taken with 2 µm width and minimum length (0.25µm drawn, 0.16µm effective) in order to improve the frequency response of this current mirror. This improvement in the current mirror frequency response allowed to increase the m factor from 6 to 10, with the consequent increase in the transconductance multiplication factor and current drive that allows us to reduce consumption. The calculated results predict a transition frequency of 12.7 MHz with 74° phase margin and 94 dB of open loop gain with a purely capacitive load of 5pF, while the consumption was reduced from 99µA in the 2 µm process down to 64 µA in the 0.25 µm. It must be pointed out that this is the result of a redesign of a 2µm design, not a design completely optimized for the 0.25µm process, in which case larger improvements might still be achievable.

4. EXPERIMENTAL RESULTS

4.1 Test Setups

Some of the test setups we applied are shown in Figure 5-7. The setup shown in Figure 5-7 a), applied in [LAN99], enables the direct measurement of the open loop high frequency response with a network analyzer (HP 4195 in our case). For low frequency gain measurements both the setups of Figure 5-7 b) and c) were applied with the HP 3563A low frequency analyzer. These setups were applied with a buffer implemented with a J-FET input TL071 commercial op amp when measurements without load resistor were required. The circuit of Figure 5-7 c) is a classical circuit for measuring the open loop gain of op amps that multiplies the small input signal to be measured by (1+R3/R4).

For settling time and frequency response measurements in amplifiers A3 and A4, an active probe with 2pF input capacitance was applied.

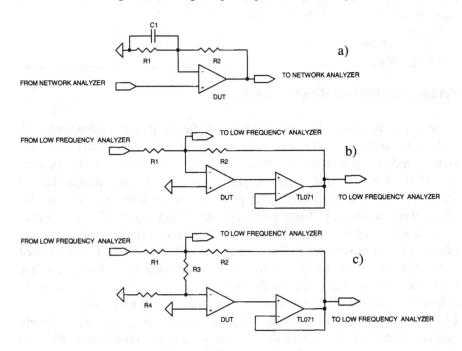

Figure 5-7. Test setups a) for transition frequency and phase margin measurements; b) and c) for low frequency gain measurements.

4.2 Measurement Data of the Amplifiers

Next, we will present the complete characterization data of amplifier A3. Then we will summarize the main results for amplifiers A1, A2 and A4. Amplifiers A1, A5 and A6 will be further discussed in the next chapter in the framework of their application to the pacemaker sense channel.

Amplifier A3 was chosen to discuss characterization data in detail since their specifications are easily comparable with those of other published amplifiers, and this amplifier is more representative of general purpose op amps than, for example, amplifier A1 whose design is very specific to the intended application.

5 MHz FD SOI Amplifier

Table 5-5 compares the characteristics of amplifier A3 that result from calculation with MATLAB, simulation with SPICE and measurements.

Table 5-5. Measured characteristics of A3 amplifier.

	Calculation	Simulation	Measurement	Notes
f_T (MHz)	5.9	6.0	5.7	C_2=8pF
PM (°)	80	75	68	C_2=8pF
A_0 (dB) @ R2=∞	98	92	87.4	C_2=8pF
A_0 (dB) @ R2=10kΩ	74		66	C_2=8pF
I_{DDq} (µA)	99	102	106	C_2=8pF
SR (output rise, V/µs)	3		1.6	1, C_2=10pF
SR (output fall, V/µs)	3		4.0	1, C_2=10pF
Total Settling time rise (ns), 5%	305		311	2, C_2=10pF
Total Settling time rise (ns), 1%	339		502	2,4, C_2=10pF
Total Settling time fall (ns), 5%	144		243	2,3, C_2=10pF
Total Settling time fall (ns), 1%	177		480	2, 3, 4, C_2=10pF
Input Common Mode Range	VSS+0.05V / VDD-0.7V		VTn=0.52V, |Vtp|=0.62V	
Output swing	VSS+0.13V / VDD-0.23V			
Minimum VDD (V)			1.5	5
Offset (mV)			22	6
THD(dB)			-64	Vo=1.2Vpp, 7
THD(dB)			-61	Vo=1.4Vpp, 7
THD(dB)			-29	Vo=1.5Vpp, 7

Notes:

In all measurements, the output stage reference current is set to 1.65µA instead of the 2µA design value to take into account the error in current mirror factors (see discussion below). Unless otherwise noted the supply voltage is 2V.

1. The calculation value of the SR corresponds to the ideal value of $2*I_{D1}/C_f$
2. The calculation value of settling times has taken into account the measured values of SR (1.6V/µs rise and 4.0V/µs fall), f_T (5.6MHz) and PM (64°) in the same load configuration as in the settling measurement. The amplifier is in follower configuration and the input step has 0.5V amplitude.
3. Fall settling much more oscillatory, see analysis below.
4. Measurements at 1% are much less reliable because the error to be measured is close to the oscilloscope quantization step.
5. Criterion to define minimum V_{DD}: value that makes the transition frequency change by 10%. The limitation is set by the biasing transistors gate-source voltage. This value can be lowered by resizing these transistors.
6. Measured in follower configuration when the settling measurement was taken.
7. Input frequency: 10kHz, closed loop gain: -1, V_{DD}=2V.

Let us discuss these results.

a) The application of minimum sized transistors in the output stage current mirrors to favor frequency response leads to noticeable errors in the copy factors due to mismatching. These errors gave a higher output stage current when the design value of the reference current was used (total current of 120µA instead of the approximately 100µA resulting from simulation and calculations). The output stage reference current (I_{refo} in Figure 5-6) applied during the measurements was adjusted so that the measured total current was equal to the calculated total current.

b) The measured open loop gain for the result shown in Table 5-5 is plotted in Figure 5-8. A small change of slope of the open loop gain amplitude is visible at the low frequency end of this plot. This is an effect introduced by the test setup of Figure 5-7 a), because at this frequency the impedance of C_1 is no longer negligible.

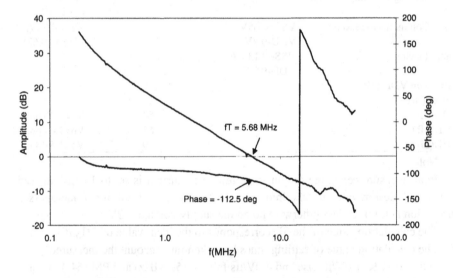

Figure 5-8. Measured open loop gain amplitude and phase of amplifier A3.

c) As described above, the procedure applied to calculate k, h, m and the non dominant pole position, which was based on the approximate phase margin expression of Eq. (5.12), leads to a design with increased phase margin. The measured phase margin was a bit smaller, probably due to the phase margin dependence on the parasitic and load capacitances which are not precisely known. Nevertheless, the measured phase margin (68°) still makes it possible to further increase the transition frequency with acceptable stability. This was experimentally done by changing the input stage reference current (I_{refi} in Figure 5-6). The result is shown in Figure 5-9. The total consumption changes very little between the amplifiers plotted in Figure 5-9, since the input stage current is a small percentage of the total consumption. Only an increase of 4μA is required to have a transition frequency of 9.9MHz with 50° phase margin.

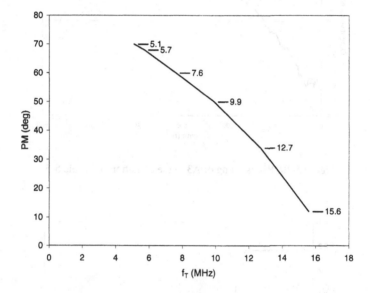

Figure 5-9. Phase margin (PM) vs. transition frequency of amplifier A3, while varying the input stage reference current.

d) The difference between the actual slew rate and the value calculated with the theoretical expression is also noticeable in simulations and is mainly due to the effect of the parasitic capacitance at the sources of the input stage transistors. This capacitance is in parallel with the "tail" current source of the input differential pair. Depending on the slope of the step, the current through this capacitor either adds or subtracts to the current of the source that determines the slew rate.

e) The rise and fall settlings measured under the conditions of Table 5-5 are shown in Figure 5-10 and Figure 5-11. The fall settling is too oscillatory for high and medium amplitude output steps. This is a consequence of the turn on delay of the current mirrors. A simple modification of the circuit architecture that improves this behavior is discussed below in Section 5.

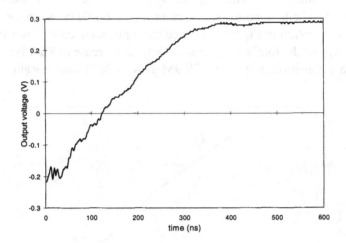

Figure 5-10. Rise settling of A3 in the conditions of Table 5-5

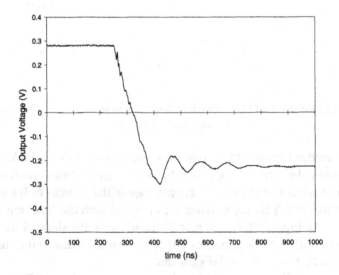

Figure 5-11. Fall settling behavior of A3 in the conditions of Table 5-5

f) The amplifier features very good voltage ranges and the minimum measured supply voltage for 10% change in the transition frequency was 1.5V. This is not the ultimate low voltage achievable by this amplifier, since in this case the limitation was due to the output stage bias current mirror M_{os1} and M_{os2} (see schematic diagram in Figure 5-6). This limit can be extended by biasing these transistors in weaker inversion. Furthermore, these results correspond to an FD SOI wafer initially intended for high temperature operation, with n and p threshold voltages around 0.5V and 0.6V. The results would be further improved in lower voltage FD SOI processes that have threshold voltages around 0.3 to 0.4V.

g) An example of the measured spectrum for determination of the total harmonic distortion is shown in Figure 5-12.

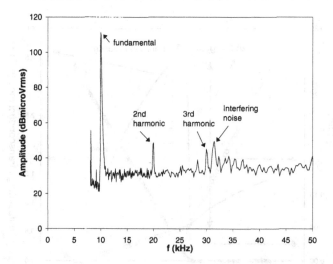

Figure 5-12. Measured spectrum for determination of total harmonic distortion of amplifier A3, in inverting amplifier configuration with gain –1, 1.4V$_{pp}$ output voltage.

This result agrees with what can be analytically estimated as follows. We consider the main source of harmonic distortion is the asymmetry of the output stage. In the closed loop gain (A_{cl}) expression of Eq. (5.1), we introduce the effect of the output stage asymmetry as a change in the second stage gain A_2, which we will represent as an average value A_{2av} multiplied by a variation term $(1+\delta A_2)$. Then the relative closed loop gain error is given by:

$$\left| \frac{A_{cl} - A_{clav}}{A_{clav}} \right| = \frac{|\delta A_2|}{1 + A_1.A_{2av}(1+\delta A_2).\beta} \tag{5.15}$$

where A_{clav} is the closed loop gain when the second stage gain equals the average value A_{2av}.

The main contribution to the variation δA_2 is the variation in the output stage transconductance, which is shown in Figure 5-13 and is related to the g_{mmult} factor. The maximum of the error given by Eq. (5.15) occurs when the A_2 gain is minimum. From Figure 5-13, the minimum A_2 gain corresponds to δA_2 (which is given by the relative deviation of the output stage transconductance from its average value) equal to -0.7. Evaluating Eq. (5.15) in this case, with $A_1.A_{2av}$ equal to the measured open loop gain (87.4dB) and β equal to one (in order to compare with the distortion that was measured in unity gain configuration), the maximum relative error equals to –69dB, which is close to the measured distortion.

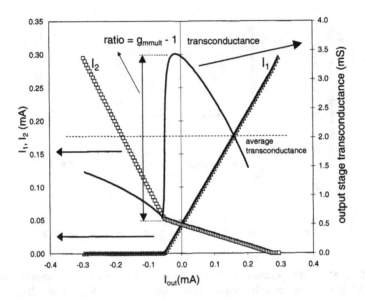

Figure 5-13. Simulated output transistor currents I_1 (pMOS, triangle symbols) and I_2 (nMOS, square symbols) and output stage transconductance (solid line) vs. output current. The average transconductance, defined as the average between the maximum and minimum value, is also shown (dashed line).

Other Experimental Prototypes

Table 5-6, Table 5-7 and Table 5-8 summarize the measurement results for amplifiers A1, A2 and A4.

Amplifier A2, as amplifier A3 did, shows an important deviation between predicted and measured total quiescent current. Through measurements of the total quiescent current as a function of the reference currents, it was verified that the origin of this difference is in the second stage current. This difference is attributed to variations in the current mirrors gain. Amplifiers A2 and A4 present, as amplifier A3 did, differences between the predicted and measured phase margin. These results suggest that the influence of parasitic capacitances and current mirror gains in the phase margin require to work with increased design margins. Letting aside these differences the amplifiers have good performance.

Table 5-6. Calculated vs. measured results for amplifier A1 at 2V supply voltage and 10nA reference current.

	Calculated	Measured
f_{T1ord} (kHz)	178	187
f_{ndp} (kHz) @ $C_2 \cong 32$ pF	39	35
A_0 (dB)	120	> 80
I_{DD} (nA)	83	89.5
V_{offset} (mV)		8.6

Table 5-7. Calculated vs. measured results for amplifier A2 for different reference current settings, 2V supply voltage and 22pF load capacitance.

Bias Currents I_{refi}, I_{refo}	$I_{refi} = 0.5\mu A$, $I_{refo} = 0.5\mu A$		$I_{refi} = 0.5\mu A$, $I_{refo} = 0.335\mu A$	$I_{refi} = 1.0\mu A$, $I_{refo} = 0.335\mu A$
	Calculated	Measured	Measured	Measured
f_T (MHz)	0.76	0.78	0.77	1.4
PM (°)	68	58	50	50
A_0 (dB)	122	-	92	-
I_{DD} (μA)	23	34	23.1	24.3
THD (dB) @ Vo=1.6Vpp, 10kHz, -1 closed loop gain				-59
THD (dB) @ Vo=1.8Vpp, 10kHz, -1 closed loop gain				-50

Table 5-8. Calculated vs. measured results for amplifier A4 for different reference current settings, 2V supply voltage and 5.5 pF load capacitance.

Bias Currents I_{refi}, I_{refo}	$I_{refi} = 1.0\mu A$, $I_{refo} = 5.0\mu A$		$I_{refi} = 0.7\mu A$, $I_{refo} = 5.0\mu A$	
	Calculated	Measured	Calculated	Measured
f_T (MHz)	14.4	13	10.4	10.5
PM (°)	74	48	74	55
A_0 (dB)	81	70	82	-
I_{DD} (μA)	103	96	102	95
THD (dB) @Vo = 1.3Vpp, 10kHz, -1 closed loop gain				-49

In order to better compare amplifiers A3 (fabricated in a 2 μm FD SOI process) and A4 (fabricated in a 0.8 μm bulk process), Figure 5-14 plots the measured phase margin versus transition frequency for amplifier A3 (previously plotted in Figure 5-9) together with those measured for amplifier A4. The total currents are approximately equal in both cases. Figure 5-14 shows an advantage for amplifier A4, but a small one, not as big as the initial design data of Table 5-1 suggested, since as already mentioned, these data corresponded to different phase margin conditions. The advantage for amplifier A4 with respect to A3, can be in part traced to a similar difference between their technologies (0.8μm bulk and 2μm SOI) in terms of parasitic capacitances. Evaluating the parasitic capacitance that sets a current mirror frequency response, for the case of a mirror implemented with 2μm/2μm transistors in the SOI technology and a mirror implemented   with 2μm/0.8μm transistors in the Bulk technology (where 2μm is the minimum width allowed by the design rules), we have a ratio of 1.15 the 2μm FD SOI capacitance over the 0.8μm Bulk capacitance. On the other hand, the A3 amplifier in FD SOI still outperforms the A4 amplifier in terms of gain, input common mode range and distortion.

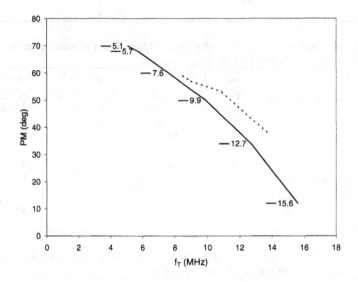

Figure 5-14. Phase margin (PM) vs. transition frequency of amplifier A3 (solid line) at 8pF load capacitance and amplifier A4 (dashed line) at 7.3pF load capacitance, while varying the input stage reference current.

Table 5-9 summarizes the calculated and measured data of amplifiers A3, A4 and the redesign of amplifier A4 for 2μm Bulk technology.

Table 5-9. Comparison of amplifiers A3, A4 and redesign of A4 for 2 μm bulk.

Amplifier	A3		A4		A4
Technology	2 μm FD SOI		0.8 μm Bulk		2.0 μm Bulk
Bias Currents (μA) I_{refi} / I_{refo}	2.0 / 2.0	2.0 / 1.65	0.7 / 5.0		1.0 / 5.0
C_2(pF)	8	8	5.5	5.5	5.5
	Calculated	Measured	Calculated	Measured	Calculated
f_T (MHz)	10.5	9.9	10.4	10.5	10.4
PM (°)	74	50	74	55	57
A_0 (dB)	96	87 (Note 1)	82	70	90
I_{DD} (μA)	99	110	102	95	243
Input Common Mode Range (V)	0.07 / 1.23 (Note 2) 0.15 / 1.51 (Note 3)	- / > 1.25 (Note 1, 2)	0.15 / 1.15	-	0.09 / 1.05
THD (dB) @ Vopp , f = 10kHz, closed loop gain –1.	-	-64 @ 1.2, -61 @ 1.4	-	-49 @ 1.3	-

Note 1: Measured at I_{refi} 1.0μA that corresponds to 5.7 MHz transition frequency.
Note 2: Measured and calculated for a process with $V_{T0n} = 0.52$V and $V_{T0p} = 0.62$V
Note 3: Calculated for a process with $V_{T0n} = 0.4$V and $V_{T0p} = 0.4$V

4.3 Comparison with other published results

In Table 5-10 and Table 5-11, amplifiers A2 and A3 are compared with published results of amplifiers with similar bandwidth.

We will briefly describe these amplifiers in order to later evaluate the comparison results. The amplifiers compared with A2 are: an amplifier for a switched capacitor circuit which applies the same class AB output stage, but without exploiting the transconductance multiplication effect that we have proposed [VER96], a four stage amplifier with nested G_m-C compensation [YOU97] and an amplifier with rail to rail input and class AB output stage [FER97].

The amplifiers compared with A3 are: a general purpose amplifier with rail-to-rail input [GRI97] and two amplifiers with class AB output stages, the first one with a standard input stage and the second one with a rail-to-rail input stage [LAN97].

The last three rows of these tables include the figures of merit discussed in Chapter 4. In analyzing the last row, which considers the theoretical limit for power consumption, it must be taken into account that only the quiescent current of the amplifier is considered, the power delivered to the load and the output stage efficiency are not considered. This index is provided as an additional element to compare the amplifiers, but is a partial comparison element. For example as the noise power is proportional to the bandwidth considered, which we reckoned to be f_T, the denominator of this index, equal to $8kTf_T.S/N$, is independent of f_T. This explains why it gives similar values for amplifier A3 and the amplifiers presented in reference [LAN97], while these ones consume more and have a smaller bandwidth.

Table 5-10. Comparison of amplifier A2 with other published amplifiers for similar transition frequency.

	A2 v1	A2 v2	[VER96]	[YOU97]	[FER97]
Technology	SOI 3μm	SOI 3μm	SOI 2.4μm	Bulk 2μm	Bulk 0.7μm
Supply voltage (V)	2	2	10	2	1.5
Quiescent supply current (μA)	24	34	60	700	307
Load resistance / capacitance	10k/22p	10k/22p	50p	10k/20p	15p
DC gain (dB) (@ load resistor)	76 (10kΩ) 92 (∞)	76 (10kΩ) 92 (∞)	100 (∞)	100 (10k)	84 (∞)
Transition frequency (MHz)	1.4	0.78	1.2	1	1.3
Phase margin (°)	50	58	60	58	64
Equivalent input noise (nV/√Hz)	35 (Note 1)	47 (Note 1)	n/a	n/a	25
Output swing (Vpp @ THD (dB))	1.8 (@ -50)	1.8 (@ -50)	n/a	1.0 (@ -70)	0.9 (@ -40)
GHz/W	17	11.5	2	0.7	2.8
GHz.pF/W	374	253	100	14	42
Quiescent supply power / (8.kT.f_T.S/N)	6.9	17.6	n/a	n/a	134

Note 1: Input noise estimated as thermal noise of input stage.

These comparisons show the advantage of the proposed architecture for low-power applications, especially in terms of significantly increased frequency/power (GHz/Watt) and (GHz.pF/Watt) ratios. The proposed architecture has lower, though acceptable, DC gain due to the low load resistances considered, but their gain significantly rises when considered with a purely capacitive load, as is the case in switched capacitor circuits.

A small part of the higher consumption in some of the compared amplifiers can be explained by the rail to rail input stage ([FER97], [GRI97] and [LAN97], second amplifier). Nevertheless, this is not sufficient to explain the more than 10 times increase of consumption as shown by amplifiers of references [FER97] and [GRI97]. Moreover, the increased input common mode range available in SOI might allow to apply an standard input stage in an application that otherwise would require a rail to rail input. An additional, larger, part of the increased consumption might come from the application of complex class AB or multistage structures in order to be able to achieve high gain with low load resistors ([YOU97], [GRI97] and [LAN97]). This is in fact one of the motivations of our architecture, to suit applications where a large current drive is not needed and minimum consumption is an essential feature. The final advantage to our amplifiers is given by the joint effects of a power conscious design, the transconductance multiplication principle and the advantages of SOI technology.

Table 5-11. Comparison of amplifier A3 with other published amplifiers for similar transition frequency.

	A3	[GRI97]	[LAN97]	[LAN97]
Technology	SOI 2μm	BiCMOS	Bulk 1.6μm	Bulk 1.6μm
Supply voltage (V)	2	1	1.8	1.8
Quiescent supply current (μA)	105	1200	180	221
Load resistance / capacitance	10kΩ/8pF	10kΩ	10kΩ/5pF	10kΩ/5pF
DC gain (dB)	66 (10kΩ)	110 (600Ω)	88 (10kΩ)	90 (10kΩ)
(@ load resistor)	87 (∞)			
Transition frequency (MHz)	7.6	4	5	5.8
PM (deg)	60	60	62	57
Equivalent input noise (nV/√Hz)	37.5	35	30	30
	(Note 1)			
Output Swing (Vpp)	1.4	0.9	1.4	1.4
GHz/Watt	36	3.8	15.4	14.6
GHz*pF/Watt	288	-	77	73
Quiescent supply power /	57	1374	56	69
$(8.kT.f_T.S/N)$				

Note 1: Input noise estimated as thermal noise of input stage.

5. IMPROVEMENTS OF DESIGN METHOD AND ARCHITECTURE

5.1 Settling behavior

The main deficiency of the architecture in a general application case is the fact that the minimum current in the output branches is not fixed. This is particularly problematic in the p –side since there we have a current mirror "chain" that leads to an important turn-on delay with the consequence of oscillatory settling when a large amplitude step is applied.

Referring to the circuit of Figure 5-4 b), the problem arises when the current through M_f reaches the I_{refAB} value, cutting off transistor M_e. Various approaches were investigated to solve this problem. Some of them tried to limit the current that is taken from the I_{refAB} source by the M_f branch. They were based on applying a circuit in series with M_f that gives as output the maximum between the current through M_f and a reference current; or limiting the current through M_f by inserting a transistor between the source of M_f and ground that is normally in the linear region and saturates to a maximum allowable current. The main difficulty is to solve the problem without jeopardizing the good frequency, power and supply voltage characteristics of the circuit. The final solution came from adapting a clamping circuit proposed in [CAS92] for avoiding cut-off of the output stage devices in buffer amplifiers. The circuit with transistors M_{11}, M_{12}, M_{13} and current source I_{bias} is added to the junction of M_e and M_f as shown in Figure 5-15. The bias circuit formed by I_{bias}, M_{12} and M_{13} is so designed that in normal conditions the current through M_{11} is negligible. When M_f conducts heavily during a transient, M_{11} limits how low the gate-source voltage of M_e gets. In the design of the circuit there is a compromise between settling improvement and loss of performance (consumption, gain, frequency) of the output stage.

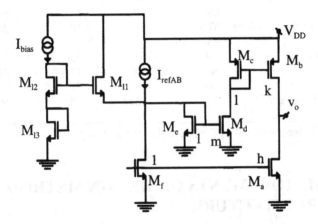

Figure 5-15. Class AB stage modification to limit cut-off of the current mirrors and improve the settling behavior in a falling step.

Figure 5-16 shows a simulation of amplifier A3 with its output stage modified with this circuit where M_{11}, M_{12} and M_{13} are all taken of small size (3µm/2µm) to favor frequency operation and I_{bias} is 3µA. The behavior during a falling step of the output voltage and gate-source voltage of M_e are shown, comparing the simulation of the original and modified designs. In the new circuit, the simulated total current consumption increases from the original 96µA to 108µA, while the transition frequency remains unchanged, the phase margin decreases from 70° to 66° and the DC gain decreases from 89 dB to 85 dB. These results, which could be further optimized by changing the sizing of the rest of the stage, show how this simple modification keeps the essential advantages of the proposed stage, while improving the settling behavior.

The main price paid for the improvement in the settling behavior is that now the minimum supply voltage of the stage is two gate-source voltage (V_{GS}) plus one drain saturation voltage (V_{DSAT}) instead of the original V_{GS} + V_{DSAT}.

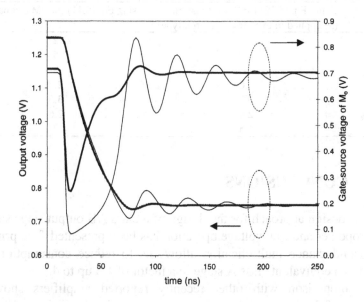

Figure 5-16. Simulation of original A3 design (light lines) and design modified according to Figure 5-15 (dark lines).

5.2 Exact calculation of the phase margin

Some improvements to the design method have been discussed previously. The first one is to apply the more exact expression of the phase margin given by Eq. (5.11) in the determination of k, h, m. Table 5-12 compares the results obtained applying this improved method to the results of the original design of amplifier A3. It is shown that the quiescent consumption can be further reduced with respect to the class A case.

In the case of amplifier A1, we could further reduce the current mirrors pole frequencies, by taking into account that the final design non dominant pole frequency is lower than the transition frequency and that a large safety margin was taken since the non dominant pole was specified 2 decades above the high −3dB frequency of the pacemaker filter (at 20kHz). The resulting values in this less conservative design are: k=16, h=2, m=4, which lead to a total consumption of 40nA, instead of the original 83nA.

Other alternatives to further improve the design method are to apply a more exact model of the current mirror poles (e.g. by considering Eq. (5.10)) and applying the optimization procedure for a given total settling time presented in Chapter 4.

Table 5-12. Comparison of design of amplifier A3 based on determination of the phase margin with Eq. (5.11) and Eq. (5.12)).

	Using Eq. (5.12) for PM estimation (as applied in experimental prototype)	Using Eq. (5.11) for PM estimation.
k	2	2
h	2	5
m	6	9
w_{ndp0}/w_T	3.6	2.2
g_{mmult}	6.1	3.5
$(g_m/I_D)_{mult}$	2.9	2.6
I_A/I_{AB}	1.5	2

6.   CONCLUSIONS

A new design approach for the design of a class AB output stage suitable for micropower and low voltage operation has been presented. The principle of transconductance multiplication allows us to reduce consumption with respect to an equivalent class A stage in a factor of 1.5 up to 4.

The comparison with other recently reported amplifiers show the advantages of this approach when power consumption is a primary concern. The advantages of SOI technology allowed us to reach comparable frequency behavior for the same total consumption in an amplifier in 2 μm SOI technology and an amplifier in a 0.8μm bulk technology, while the gain, distortion and input common mode range were improved in the SOI case.

The requirements for the OTA of the pacemaker sense channel are satisfied in an experimental prototype with a total quiescent current of 83nA. This consumption could be further reduced to 40nA in a design based on an exact calculation of the amplifier phase margin.

Chapter 6

Implementation of Pacemaker Sense Circuits

This chapter describes the design of pacemaker sense circuits, taking advantage of various techniques and ideas developed in this book. Two experimental realizations are presented. First we describe a switched capacitor (SC) design of the sense channel filter / amplifier in 0.8μm Bulk technology. Then, we present the continuous time implementation in FD SOI technology, applying the general architecture described in Chapter 2 [SIL021].

1. SWITCHED CAPACITOR FILTER / AMPLIFIER IMPLEMENTATION

The motivations for the design of this SC version of sense channel filter/amplifier are twofold. On the one hand, we seek to test the application of the class AB amplifier architecture studied in Chapter 5 to a switched capacitor circuit. On the other hand, we want to explore the trade-offs involved in a switched capacitor implementation of this kind of circuit. Specifically, we discuss the difficulties encountered due to the high gain required and the design criteria adopted to overcome these difficulties, while reducing power consumption.

A first comment is due on the issue of the switches operation at 2V. As discussed in Chapter 3, in standard bulk technologies, it is not possible to have switches that operate with low resistance in the whole range of a 2 V power supply. This is indeed the case for supply voltages below 2.8V in the 0.8μm process used here, considering the nominal threshold voltage values. This problem is usually circumvented either boosting the clock signal voltages above V_{DD} or applying the switched op amp technique [CRO94] as is done in the switched capacitor based sense channel presented in [GER012]. Nevertheless, if we keep the overall sense channel architecture discussed in Chapters 1 and 2, where we apply, as quiescent DC voltage for the filter and amplifier, 7/32 of V_{DD}, most of the switches operate outside of the "gap" in the switch conductance. The problem remains for some of the switches connected to the output of the filter if we want the output to be able to swing across the half V_{DD} range, as happened in the original design. This can be solved by reducing the output range and then programming the detection thresholds by a combination between the D/A values and the gain of the filter, which can be easily programmed in a switched capacitor implementation. This is in fact the approach taken in reference [LEN01] and the one we will assume here.

The consumption of a switched capacitor circuit is directly related to the consumption of their operational amplifiers, which is determined by the required transition frequency. We will now summarize the criteria to fix the transition frequency of the operational amplifiers. Classical works on this issue ([TEM80, MAR81, GRE86]) derive the expression of the error due to finite gain-bandwidth in a general case, but they focus on simplified expressions for the derivation of design criteria. These simplified expressions do not apply when the stage is intended to provide voltage gain. Therefore, the popular rule of setting the amplifier transition frequency to be five times the clock frequency ([MAR81, GRE86]) applies for "pure" filters with unity gain in the pass band. However, it does not apply in some of the amplifiers of the kind of circuits we are considering, which are intended to provide high gain together with the filtering function.

We will illustrate this by considering the inverting integrator of Figure 6-1, which will be providing the gain in our biquad filter. We will consider that the ideal frequency response of the filter $H_i(e^{jwT})$, with T the clock period and w the angular frequency, is related to the real frequency response $H(e^{jwT})$ by:

$$H\left(e^{jwT}\right) = \frac{H_i\left(e^{jwT}\right)}{1 - m(w) - j\theta(w)} \tag{6.1}$$

The effect of the finite amplifier bandwidth (represented in the following equations by w_T, the transition angular frequency), leads to the following error factors [GRE86]:

$$m(w) = -e^{-k_1}[1 - k.\cos(wT)]$$

$$\theta(w) = -e^{-k_1}.k.\sin(wT) \qquad (6.2)$$

$$k = \frac{1}{1+\dfrac{C_1}{C_2}}, \quad k_1 = k.w_T.T/2$$

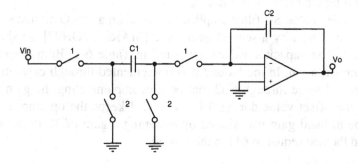

Figure 6-1. Inverting SC integrator for analysis of influence of finite op amp bandwidth.

Let us analyze these expressions. We are usually interested in the behavior of the filter for frequencies much smaller than the clock frequency, i.e. the product w.T is much smaller than one. Then, sin(w.T) is small. On the other hand, the gain in the integrator of Figure 6-1, as well as in the biquad implemented with this integrator, is proportional to C_1/C_2. Hence, if we aim at a filter with high gain (in the pacemaker sense channel we need an in band gain in the 600 to 700 range), the factor k defined above will be small. In this case the error term $\theta(w)$ will be negligible and the error m(w) will be given by:

$$m(w) \cong -e^{-k_1} \qquad (6.3)$$

As w_T appears in this expression multiplied by k, an increase on the gain requires an equal increase of the transition frequency to keep a constant error. This is in fact a consequence of the constant gain bandwidth product of a closed loop amplifier. If we aim at 1% error (m(w) = 0.01), with a gain of 600, this requires k_1 to be 4.6 and the transition frequency must relate to the clock frequency f_{CLK} by:

$$f_T = \frac{k_1}{k.\pi}f_{CLK} = \frac{k_1}{\pi}\left(1+\frac{C_1}{C_2}\right)f_{CLK} = 880.f_{CLK} \;\;!!! \qquad (6.4)$$

If we add this to the fact that the clock frequency must be much larger than the signal bandwidth to ease the anti alias filter design, we get to an extremely inefficient situation. This imposes the need for implementing the gain in several stages to optimize this gain-bandwidth trade off, a well known strategy in analog circuit design. To share the gain in several stages also helps in decreasing the capacitor spread required to implement the circuit. On the other hand to have more than one gain stage brings up the issues of either decoupling the DC component between them or compensating the offset of the stages.

The implemented SC filter-amplifier is based on a low Q biquad structure [GRE86], followed by a second gain stage [MAR87, JOH97], as shown in Figure 6-2. The capacitor values are listed in Table 6-1. Both stages have offset compensation. In the biquad it is implemented through capacitor CI2. In the second stage through Ca2 that besides implementing the gain factor, samples the offset value during $\Phi 1$, while Ca3 keeps the op amp in closed loop. The in-band gain was shared by assigning a gain of 10 to the second stage and the rest (equal to 61) to the biquad.

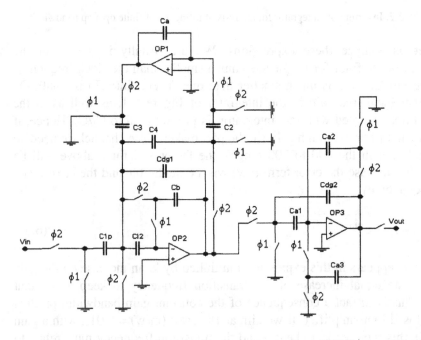

Figure 6-2. Schematic diagram of pacemaker sense channel SC filter/amplifier.

Table 6-1. Capacitor values in pF.

C2, C4, Ca2, Ca3	C3	C1p	Ca	Cb, Cl2	Ca1	Cdg1, Cdg2	Total Capacitance
1	2.25	61	66.25	5.5	10	0.25	155

Additional measures taken to reduce consumption were the following:

a) The biquad structure was organized so that OP1 and OP2 settled in different clock phases. The results previously described for the influence of the amplifier f_T assumed that the input of the stage was a sample and held signal, which would not be the case if the amplifiers were obliged to settle in cascade during the same clock phase.

b) In the gain stage, that will be the one handling the bigger signals, the applied structure, besides compensating offset, has the additional benefit of keeping the output from going to zero in any of the phases. This is due to the action of Ca3 that samples the output voltage during $\Phi 1$ and maintains it during $\Phi 2$. This helps to reduce consumption by much reducing the slew rate requirement on OP3. This effect is reinforced by the presence of the "deglitching" capacitors ([MAT87, JOH97]) Cdg1 and Cdg2 that keep the op. amps. fedback during the non overlapping period of the clock phases, thus avoiding output glitches.

The clock frequency was chosen so that a simple first order passive RC circuit with low precision, feasible in integrated form, would be sufficient as antialias filter. It was taken at 10kHz, i.e. 50 times the band edge of 200Hz. For this clock frequency, the analysis of the influence of the op amp bandwidth with expressions as the ones described above, for 1 % error, leads to a requirement of an f_T of at least 150kHz for OP2. For amplifier OP1, an f_T of only about 1kHz is required, in the final design a value much higher than this (40kHz) was applied. Slew rate is not a limiting factor in this case due to the measures taken at the architectural level.

The same amplifier cell as the one applied for OP2 was applied for OP3, trading off a small consumption reduction for reduced design time.

The amplifiers were designed with the architecture presented in Chapter 5.

The theoretical consumption of amplifier OP2 is 400nA and for amplifier OP1 it is 190nA, giving a total consumption of 990nA. The measured consumption was 1.4μA. This large deviation is explained because the mirrors that copy the reference current of the class AB output stage from the bias current reference are not made based on unitary transistors but with, for example in the case of amplifier OP2, transistors of sizes 2μm / 20μm and 7.7 μm / 20μm. The influence of the effective width was taken into account during the design, but there is another effect that is equally important: the variation of threshold voltage with the transistor width. In this process the typical threshold voltage decreases by 30mV from a 2/20 transistor to a 20/20 transistor. Such a change in threshold voltage, in weak inversion is translated to a change in current of:

$$\Delta I = e^{\frac{\Delta V_{TO}}{n.U_T}} \tag{6.5}$$

which corresponds to a doubling of the current for ΔV_{TO} of 30mV, n equal to 1.5 and 26mV room temperature U_T. In our case, though the change in transistor width is smaller a 13mV change in V_{TO} is enough for explaining the measured change in quiescent current. This difference can be easily corrected by copying the current with multiple parallel unitary transistors.

Figure 6-3 plots the measured frequency responses at 2V together with the ideal target response. The result of a Switcap simulation is coincident with the ideal target response. The measured frequency response at 2.8V is practically identical to the 2V response.

To finish, we will compare this circuit to other switched capacitor implementations of pacemaker sense channel found in the literature. We will consider for the comparison the theoretical consumption value of 1μA, since the deviation in the measured current can be corrected using multiple unitary transistors for the bias current mirror layout.

In references [GER012] and [LEN01] results are presented for pacemaker sense channels based on SC circuits, both also in a 0.8μm bulk CMOS process. Reference [GER012] presents simulation results of a channel based on a preamplifier and an SC biquad. The total current consumption is 1.3μA. In reference [LEN01] the channel is implemented with a preamplifier and a third order SC filter: first order high pass section plus second order bandpass, this last one implemented with a biquad. The total current consumption is 600nA: 450nA in the pre-amplifier and 150nA in the SC filter. It is important to note that in both of these works a first order antialiasing filter (implemented in the preamplifier) and a clock frequency of 2048 Hz (instead of the 10kHz applied in our circuit) are applied. If we would apply this 5 times smaller clock frequency, we would be able to sensibly reduce the consumption. However, the decision of reducing the clock frequency and hence accept a higher level of aliasing components is dependent on system level estimations of the expected amplitude of out of band interference. By accepting this higher interference level, a much smaller consumption is achievable.

Therefore, we can conclude that the performance of our design is comparable to or better than that of other state of the art implementations.

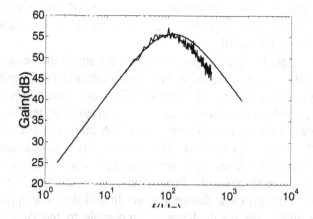

Figure 6-3. Frequency response of SC sense channel filter/amplifier: measured (solid line) and ideal target filter response (dashed line).

2. SOI CONTINUOUS TIME IMPLEMENTATION

The amplifier A1 described in Chapter 5 was applied together with a comparator to implement the continuous time sense channel architecture described for the Bulk pacemaker chip in Chapter 2. The architecture tested in SOI is shown in Figure 6-4.

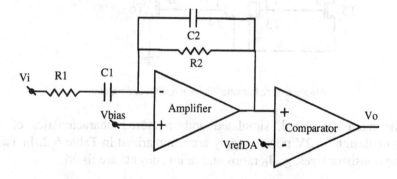

Figure 6-4. Continuous time sense channel architecture tested in SOI.

2.1 Comparator

The comparator is easily implemented with a symmetrical OTA [LAK94] followed by two inverters, as shown in Figure 6-5. The low threshold voltage of 0.5V of the SOI technology and operation in weak inversion allow us to achieve the required input range (0.44V to 1.44V) when operating from a 2V power supply with this simple structure, instead of a more complex and power hungry rail to rail structure that was required in the Bulk CMOS design of Chapter 2 [BAR96].

The design target for the comparator was to approach the design value of 15.5µs delay with an input step of 100mV amplitude and 15mV overdrive of the bulk comparator of Chapter 2. This specification corresponds to a delay of about 250µs when considering as input a triangular test signal with amplitude equal to the minimum step of the D/A converter (62.5mV at 2V power supply) and 1.5mV overdrive. This value has still a large margin from the 0.5ms maximum delay specified for the comparator, but it must be taken into account that the slope of the input signal to the comparator is further decreased due to the previous filtering stage. In addition, the application of this criterium makes the result directly comparable to the Bulk design of Chapter 2.

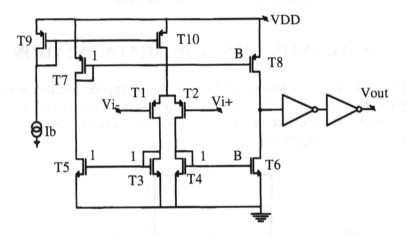

Figure 6-5. Schematic diagram of SOI comparator.

The main calculated, simulated and measured characteristics of the resulting design, at 2V power supply are summarized in Table 6-2. In Table 6-3 the transistor sizes, g_m/I_D ratios and drain currents are listed.

Table 6-2. Results of MATLAB calculations, SPICE simulations and measurements of the comparator characteristics for 2V power supply, 5nA reference current and 50 pF load. See below for comments and exact definitions of some of the magnitudes included in this table.

Magnitude	Calculation	Simulation	Measurement	Comments
Quiescent Current (nA)	15	18	19	At zero comparator output
OTA Maximum Current (nA)	40	-	-	
OTA Delay (µs)	14	28	-	100mV input step with 15mV overdrive
Total Delay (µs)	-	27.7	30.5	100mV input step with 15mV overdrive
Offset (mV)	8	-	12 (max)	Measurement maximum value in the 0.44 – 1.8V input range
Input Common Mode Range (V)	0.24-1.5	-	0.4 to > 1.5	See Note 1

Note 1. The input common mode range calculation was done considering the threshold voltages of n and p transistors are equal to 0.4V in absolute value. In the fabrication batch of the measured prototype threshold voltages varies between 0.3 and 0.5 for both n and p transistors. Since the lower limit of the input common mode range depends on the difference between the gate source voltage of the p input transistors and the n current mirror transistor, this might explain the difference between calculation and measurement in this value.

Table 6-3. Design values of transistor sizes, g_m/I_D ratios and drain currents of SOI sense channel comparator.

Transistors	W/L (µm)	g_m/I_D (1/V)	I_D (nA)
T1, T2	16.5 / 3	33	5
T3, T4, T5	3 / 71.5	20	5
T6	4 x 3 / 71.5	20	20
T7	3.5 / 30	20	5
T8	4 x 3.5 / 30	20	5
T9	7.5 / 6	30	5
T10	2 x 7.5 / 6	30	10

Several comments are due on these results.

a) The first row of the table (OTA quiescent current), refers to the consumed current in the quiescent state of the comparator in normal operation, where the comparator output is zero. In this condition, transistors T1, T3, T5, T7 and T8 (see Figure 6-5) are off and the total consumption is three times the reference current (the input reference current plus two times the reference current in the differential pair tail current source). The quiescent current of the output inverters is negligible as well as their dynamic consumption for the expected switching rate of once per cardiac cycle.

b) The second row refers to the maximum consumption of the OTA when the output is not saturated.

c) The OTA delay is measured from the point when the inputs are equal to the point where the OTA output reaches half V_{DD}. The difference between the simulated and calculated value mainly comes from the fact that a small signal linear model was applied to calculate the delay.

d) The total delay is defined from the point where the inputs are equal to the point when the comparator output reaches half V_{DD}. In the experimental measurement, the measured offset voltage was taken into account in order to have an actual 15mV overdrive, i.e. we applied at one input a step with 15mV overdrive with respect to the voltage at the other input plus the offset voltage. The delay of the output inverters is much smaller than the OTA delay (about one tenth). The fact that the total simulated delay is smaller than the simulated OTA delay is due to the fact that the delays are measured up to when half V_{DD} is crossed and the inverter threshold is smaller than half V_{DD} since the output inverters have equally sized n and p transistors. Hence, the comparator output reaches half V_{DD} before the OTA output reaches half V_{DD}.

e) The maximum measured offset voltage is a bit above the 10mV limit specified in Chapter 2. However, it should be pointed out that there is still room for improvement at the layout level: we did not apply a common centroid structure for the input differential, neither did we use dummy transistors to equalize etching effects at the sides of the current mirrors. In addition, we are not using an industrial process.

How do these results compare with those of bulk technology ? In bulk technology a rail-to-rail architecture as the one applied in Chapter 2 is required. This is so because the common mode input voltage V_{cm} is limited to:

$$V_{cm} < V_{DD} - V_{GS1,2} - V_{DSSAT10} \tag{6.6}$$

where $V_{GS1,2}$ is the gate source voltage of the transistors of the input differential pair and $V_{DSSAT10}$ is the drain source saturation voltage of the transistor T10 that implements the "tail" current source of the differential pair (see Figure 6-5). Even working deep in weak inversion, in order to achieve the required 1.44V maximum common mode voltage, a threshold voltage of no more than about 0.5V is required, which is not the case in bulk technologies. The need for a rail-to-rail architecture implies at least to double the consumption. In fact, the increase is more than twice the consumption because in the worst case for speed, when only one half of the circuit is active, it must drive, at the node where the n and p input sections join, its parasitic capacitance plus the parasitic capacitance of the other half of the rail to rail structure.

We designed a bulk rail-to-rail version of the OTA, with the architecture described in Chapter 2, which is based on a n-input and a p-input OTA connected in parallel. We kept the same gain factor of the current mirrors of the output transistors as in the SOI prototype (equal to 4). We applied the set of technology parameters, which were described in Chapter 3, corresponding to a bulk technology comparable with our SOI technology. This design needed a bias drain current through the transistors of the input differential pairs of 40nA to achieve the same calculated delay as the SOI design. In the evaluation of the output parasitic capacitances of both the SOI and bulk cases, the particular layout of the drain regions of the SOI prototype was considered for both cases, in order to make a fair comparison. This is relevant since in both cases the unitary transistors that compose the output transistors have a width that is close to the minimum of the technology, in order to minimize the output capacitance. Then the particular layout of the drain areas has more influence on the resulting parasitic capacitances.

The rail-to-rail bulk OTA has a quiescent consumption (at zero output and without considering the bias current branch) of six times this current (two times in the p-input OTA plus 4 times in the n-input OTA). This is so because in the n-input OTA, in quiescent condition, at zero output voltage, the branch corresponding to T5 and T7 in Figure 6-5 is conducting the total tail current of the differential pair. This makes a quiescent consumption without considering the bias current branch of 240nA, 12 times the equivalent quiescent consumption of the SOI prototype.

This increase in current is due to the joint effect of the following factors:
a) double circuit to have rail to rail operation, each one with the double load capacitance, since in this case the load capacitance is mainly determined by the parasitic output capacitances of the OTA (the gate capacitance of the minimum sized inverter transistors are negligible) plus,
b) the additional n-input OTA, conducts in quiescent condition 4 times the bias current of each transistor of the differential pair instead of 2 times for the p-input OTA.
c) increased load capacitance in bulk, plus
d) smaller transistor g_m/I_D ratio.

The drain current of the input differential pair of this bulk design is the same order of magnitude as the one applied in the bulk design described in Chapter 2 (50nA current through the differential pair transistors).

2.2 Experimental results of continuous time sense channel

Figure 6-6 and Figure 6-7 show the experimental performance of the SOI sense channel. In Figure 6-6 the responses of the amplifier and comparator are shown when an input test signal of 0.4mV, which is twice the minimum threshold amplitude, is applied. Figure 6-7 shows how the circuit systematically detects an input test signal of the minimum threshold amplitude of 0.2mV.

The measured output noise of the filter / amplifier is 10.4mVrms.

2.3 Overall evaluation of the continuous time implementation

The overall operation of the circuit for the detection of cardiac test signals was successfully tested. The application of a simple architecture based on power efficient building blocks, like the class AB amplifier described in Chapter 5, together with the superior characteristics of FD SOI technology made it possible to achieve an ultra low current consumption of 110nA (90 nA in the filter/amplifer and 20 nA in the comparator). This is an order of magnitude reduction with respect to previous implementations, either ours described in Chapter 2 or, for example, the one described in reference [LEN01] as well as those described in other prior works discussed in Chapter 1.

This consumption could be further reduced to only 60nA by applying the optimized design of the amplifier described in section 5.2 of Chapter 5.

The characteristics of the FD SOI technology allowed us to simplify the comparator structure and achieve an order of magnitude reduction in its consumption with respect to an implementation in a comparable bulk technology and the actual implementation presented in Chapter 2.

The main reduction in the consumption of the filter / amplifier comes from the advantages provided by the proposed class AB architecture. Here the reduction is about 6 times when compared with our industrial implementation of Chapter 2 or the filter amplifier of reference [LEN01], which consumes 450nA in the preamplifier and 150nA in the switched capacitor filter section. Here the impact of the application of the FD SOI technology is to provide a reduction of consumption of about 23% with respect a similar design implemented in bulk technology. The reduction is much smaller than the ones achieved in other circuits discussed in this book because the main consumption of this amplifier is in the output stage and this consumption is determined by the load current requirements and not by the non dominant pole position. Hence the reduction of parasitic capacitances of SOI has less effect on the total amplifier consumption.

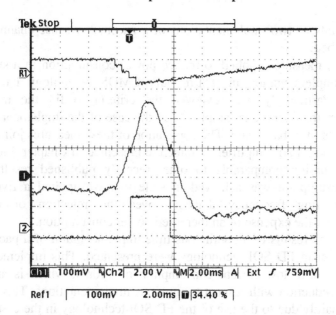

Figure 6-6. Input signal (top), filter output (middle) and comparator output (bottom). The input signal is divided by 201 prior to entering the circuit. From [SIL021], © 2002 IEEE.

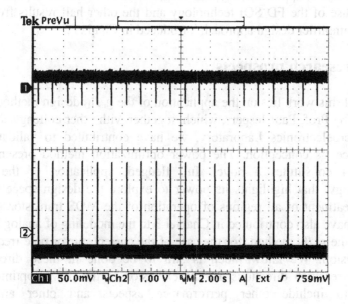

Figure 6-7. Input signal (top) and comparator output (bottom). From [SIL021], © 2002 IEEE.

3.   CONCLUSIONS AND FUTURE RESEARCH
PROSPECTS

The results of two implementations of a pacemaker sense channel have been described.

First, the measures applied to reduce power consumption in a switched capacitor implementation in 0.8µm bulk CMOS technology have been presented. Particularly, we reviewed the criteria to fix the transition frequency of the operational amplifiers in the case of the implementation of filters with high in-band gain. The application of these measures jointly with the efficient class AB amplifier architecture presented in Chapter 5 lead to a total consumption comparable to other recently published results. This similar consumption was achieved in spite that we applied a five times higher sampling frequency that improves the rejection of aliasing components at the expense of an increased power consumption.

Finally, the results of a continuous time implementation of a pacemaker sense channel in FD SOI technology were presented. This implementation achieved an ultra low current consumption of 110nA, which is an order magnitude reduction with respect to previous implementations. This current saving is mainly due to the use of the FD SOI technology in the case of the comparator and is mainly due to the application of the novel approach to the design of the class AB output stage in the case of the amplifier. Considering the whole block, approximately half of the reduction in consumption stems from the use of the FD SOI technology and the other half results from the class AB amplifier design approach introduced in Chapter 5.

Future research prospects

Most of this work lies on the application of the g_m/I_D design methodology proposed by Prof. Paul Jespers, which, together with other colleagues of the UCL Microelectronics Laboratory, we have contributed to validate and apply since its conception. The power optimization method presented in Chapter 4 constitutes a novel, full fledged, application of the g_m/I_D methodology, that highlights its power to explore the design space with a unified treatment of all regions of operation of the MOS transistor. In this work we have also contributed in Chapter 3 to the modeling of analog blocks based on the g_m/I_D method, for the case of the current mirror pole frequency and precision. We know much is still to be done in these directions. Particular research directions are the extension of the power optimization method to include other performance aspects and other amplifier architectures (particularly the class AB amplifiers described in this book). We feel this OTA design method based on power optimization could provide an interesting contribution to the advancement of the much needed and slowly advancing field of analog design automation, particularly in the field of power critical systems.

The class AB stage design approach can still be further developed and applied. One aspect is the experimental validation of the circuit modification proposed to improve the transient response. Another line of work is the application of this output stage to amplifiers with rail-to-rail input stages.

Finally, concerning the field of active medical implantable devices, we have just considered one aspect of the problem, that of the analog signal processing circuits. Additional work is needed to fully exploit the advantages of SOI in a complete pacemaker chip. Several promising prospects exist here, for example in regard to the digital circuitry, which takes an important portion of the total consumption. The voltage multiplier and polarity switches also require careful consideration. On the one hand, the absence of latch up and of connection to the common substrate of the CMOS SOI structure could greatly simplify the design of this module. On the other hand, the reduced drain-source breakdown voltage of FD SOI transistors calls for the application of special solutions in these switches that must withstand up to three times the power supply voltage (i.e. 8.4V). These solutions could probably come by way of the application of structures specifically intended for SOI [GAO92] or techniques developed to deal with the low breakdown voltage of deep sub micron bulk MOS transistors [REY97].

Concerning more general implantable applications, the demonstrated benefits of FD SOI technology in terms of reduced power consumption will grow in significance as implantable devices increase the number of measured signals and their processing in order to act more precisely on the physiological systems.

Appendix 1

Integration of Large Time Constants

This appendix details the evaluation of the components needed for implementing large time constants as well as a review of the published techniques to ease their integration.

We considered, as example for the analysis, the time constant associated to the low frequency, high pass characteristic of the sense channel filter. This time constant corresponds approximately to 70Hz, i.e. $(1/2.\pi.70)$, which is equal to 2.3ms.

We analyzed the four circuit techniques shown in Figure A1-1: an active RC filter, a MOSFET-C filter, where the resistor is implemented by the linear region resistance of a MOSFET, a transconductance – C (g_m-C) filter and a switched capacitor filter.

In the MOSFET-C technique (Figure A1-1, b)), a p-MOS transistor, which would give the highest resistance since its mobility is lower, was considered. The process data applied was the following typical data for a 2μm Bulk CMOS technology: mobility times oxide capacitance per unit area: $\mu.C_{ox} = 20\mu A/V^2$, zero source–bulk threshold voltage $V_{t0} = 0.85V$ and body-effect coefficient n of 1.5. The gate-bulk voltage applied is supposed equal to the nominal power supply voltage of 2.8V to give a high linear operation range. The DC level in the MOSFET resistor (i.e. the source-bulk voltage) is considered to be one fourth the power supply voltage, which is the actual design value in the sense channel case, which allows proper biasing for the operational amplifier and comparator.

A g_m/I_D ratio of 25V^{-1} is considered for the g_m-C filter since this is the typical value in the weak inversion region for a Bulk CMOS technology. The weak inversion region is considered since this would probably be the case at these low currents. Usually smaller g_m/I_D ratios will result from the application of techniques aiming at increasing the input linear range of the

175

transconductor; these techniques are discussed below when the methods for easing the implementation of large time constants are considered.

The sampling frequency of the switched capacitor implementation is considered at 10kHz which is fifty times the upper cut-off frequency of 200Hz to allow for a low order anti-alias filtering.

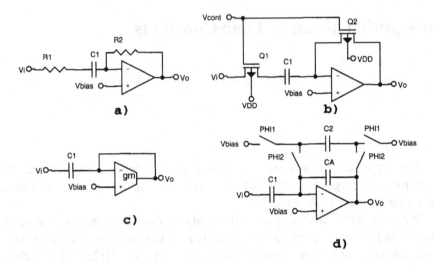

Figure A1-1. First order, high pass filtering sections considered for evaluation of feasibility of implementation of large time constants. a) Active RC, b) MOSFET-C, c) g_m-C and d) switched capacitors architectures.

If we limit the capacitance value to 100pF as a maximum value that could be integrated, then Table A1-1 shows the required value of: (1) resistance (R) for a RC filter, (2) transistor aspect ratio (W/L) for a MOSFET-C filter, (3) transconductance (g_m) and bias current required for a g_m-C filter and (4) the capacitor ratio required in a switched capacitor (SC) filter.

Table A1-1. Required components characteristics for RC, MOSFET-C, g_m-C and SC implementation of filter with time constant τ of 2.3ms and capacitor C of 100pF. The following conditions are considered: a pMOS transistor, which provides the highest resistance due to lower mobility, in the MOSFET-C filter; a typical transconductance to drain current ratio (g_m/I_D) of 25 for the g_m-C filter and a sampling frequency of 10kHz for the switched capacitor filter.

R-C filter	MOSFET-C filter	g_m–C filter		SC filter
$R = \tau/C$	$(W/L) = (R.\mu.C_{ox}.$ $\lvert(V_{GB}-V_{t0}-n.V_{SB})\rvert)^{-1}$	$g_m = 1/R$	$I_{bias} = g_m/(g_m/I_D)$	$(C_2/C_1) = \tau.f_s$
23 MΩ	(1 / 414)	43 nS	1.7 nA	23

As discussed in Chapter 2, this table shows that this time constant value is at the acceptable limit of integrated solutions or beyond it, except for the case of the switched capacitor technique. It is even more difficult to achieve an integrable solution if the stage must provide a high in-band gain, as in the case of the sense channel application.

Our solution was to implement the time constants based on external components, after considering the known alternatives for easing the implementation of large time constants. We review these techniques in the following paragraphs.

In g_m-C architectures, different approaches for decreasing the resulting transconductance to very low values with not so low bias current values have been proposed. The bias current that can be applied is limited by aspects like noise and leakage currents but also by its effect on the stage slew-rate. In evaluating the proposed solutions, attention must be paid to the effect on slew-rate, parasitic poles as for example the one associated with the current mirror that acts as active load of the differential pair and input offset voltage, since the reduction in transconductance makes that the input offset voltage due to current mismatches is increased. The techniques include: emitter degeneration, current division [RUS72], cancellation of currents components in a differential pair [GAR77] and emitter degeneration by a MOSFET operated in the triode region combined with current division [SIL97]. Furthermore in reference [SAR97] four techniques for extending the linear range of a transconductor are described. These techniques also result in lowering its transconductance.

The implementation of large time constants in an SC environment implies to slow down the basic filtering function of integration. One way to accomplish this is with a T-cell capacitor network [SAN84] which can be viewed either as a way of reducing the effective input capacitance to the integrator, or as a way to reduce the input voltage through a capacitive divider previous to integration. A solution along the same basic principle, is proposed in [NAG89]. This last solution is parasitic insensitive and is based on applying a single capacitor for input attenuation and integration. A different approach allows the application of a lower sampling rate without compromising the requirements imposed on the anti-alias filter by the application of a decimation filter at the input. This decimation filter is clocked at a higher rate than the rest of the filter [VON82].

Finally, capacitor multiplication methods exist to simulate a bigger capacitor value from a smaller actual one. Some of these circuits are based on the combination of a capacitor and a voltage or current amplifier [STO891]. Alternatively, reference [CUP79] proposes a method applying backward Euler integration with sampled data that leads to large capacitors simulation, based on resistor ratios, which could be also implemented as switched capacitors.

Appendix 2

Design of Accelerometer Signal Conditioning Circuit of Industrial Pacemaker IC in Bulk CMOS Technology

1. GENERAL CIRCUIT ARCHITECTURE

The main definitions of the overall architecture of the accelerometer signal conditioning circuit stem from the kind of sensor applied. It is a piezoresistive sensor based on a resistor bridge, where the voltage at the output, resulting from the unbalance of the bridge, is proportional to the acceleration. Some essential issues influencing the design are the following ([ICS00]):
- The bridge resistors have a typical value of 3.5kΩ and a range of variation from 2.5kΩ to 6.5kΩ
- The sensitivity, which is proportional to the supply voltage of the bridge, ranges from 8mV/g to 20mV/g at 5V power supply.
- The sensor passband starts at DC. Therefore, it will also sense the constant g acceleration due to gravity, depending on the sensor (person) orientation. This constant acceleration value plus the sensor offset, will result in a DC component at the sensor output that is much greater than the signal to be measured, which starts at 7mg and goes up to 340mg. From these sensor characteristics, it results that:
1. the sensor cannot be permanently powered since the required consumption is in the mA range,
2. the minimum input signal to be measured is dependent on the supply voltage of the bridge, but in any case, it is in the range of a few μVs,

3. a mechanism to get rid of the high DC component while preserving the low noise characteristics and low frequency response (0.5 to 7Hz) must be applied.

The strategy applied to reach the required consumption was based on turning the sensor on only during short time intervals necessary to sample its differential output and then process in continuous time the sampled and held signal [ARN98]. In this way the sensor is only turned on with a very small duty cycle (0.38 %) resulting in a drastic power reduction (consumption is divided by 260). An analysis technique was developed for the sizing of the sample and hold switches taking into account the effect of the switch on-resistance and leakage current [ARN97]. The main ideas and results associated to this technique, which has a broader field of application, will be presented later in this section.

Figure A2-1 shows the module's block diagram, which follows what was presented in section 2.3 of Chapter 1. Figure A2-2 depicts the sensor sampling and processing stage. The control clocks Ψ_1 and Ψ_2 are active in the low logical level and have very low duty cycle: 1/256 for Ψ_1 and 1/128 for Ψ_2.

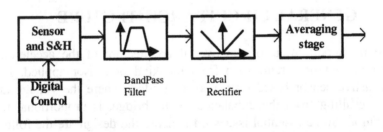

Figure A2-1. Accelerometer conditioning circuit block diagram. The blocks shown are (from left to right): sensor and sample and hold with digital control logic; 0.5 to 7Hz bandpass filter, amplifier; ideal rectifier in order to add the effect of positive and negative accelerations and a stage that performs the three seconds average to output the indicator applied for rate adaptation. From [ARN98], © 1998 IEEE.

2. IMPLEMENTATION OF THE DIFFERENTIAL INPUT BAND-PASS FILTER / AMPLIFIER

The required band-pass characteristic, which removes the input DC component, is based on a differential input amplifier with low-pass characteristic, fed back with an integrator stage that gives the high-pass characteristic. Since the input signal coming from the sensor's resistor bridge is a differential signal, the selected filter architecture must provide a differential signal input and an additional input for connection of the integrating feedback stage. The selected architecture is based on the differential difference amplifier concept [SAC87], implemented with a double input symmetrical OTA (i.e. with two input differential pairs in parallel). One input differential pair is applied for the sensor signal and the second one is applied for the integrator feedback and for the feedback network that sets the gain of the stage. A simplified schematic diagram of the stage is shown in Figure A2-3 while the double input symmetrical OTA is shown in Figure A2-4. A second gain stage, based on A3, R3, R4 and C3 is included to enhance the overall closed loop gain.

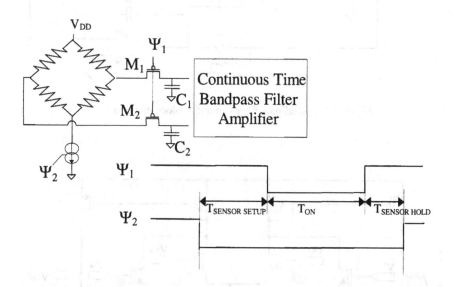

Figure A2-2. Sensor sampling and processing for reduced power consumption. When Ψ_1 is low (T_{ON}), the M_1 and M_2 switches are on and the output of the sensor is sampled on C_1, C_2. Ψ_2 controls the current through the bridge. Ψ_2 low turns the bridge on. The bridge is on a setup time ($T_{SENSOR\ SETUP}$) before T_{ON} and remains on a hold time after T_{ON}.

For analog reasons as those explained in Section 1.2 of Chapter 2, the time constants of the band pass filter were implemented through external components.

Previously an architecture based on the instrumentation amplifier presented in [STE87] was applied, as described in [ARN98]. In this architecture, the gain from the feedback input to the output is lower than the gain from the signal input. The effect is a reduction on the input offset range that can be compensated through the integrator action, whose output is bound to the power supply range. The architecture of Figure A2-4 improves this defect.

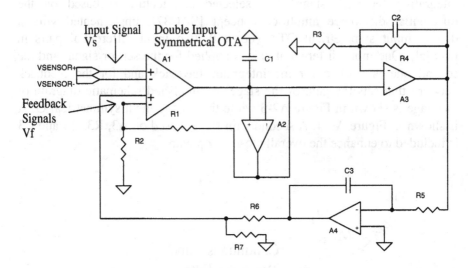

Figure A2-3. Band-pass filter / amplifier block diagram.

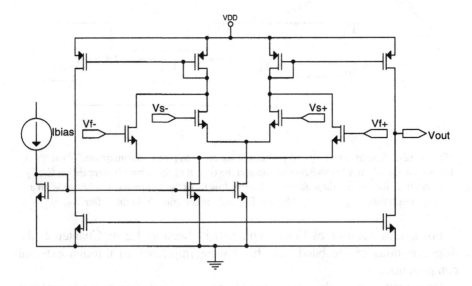

Figure A2-4. Double input symmetrical OTA that provides a differential signal input and an additional differential input for feedback purposes.

3.   RECTIFIER STAGE AND AVERAGING STAGE

The rectifier stage was implemented based on the application of switches
to change the configuration of an amplifier circuit from inverting to non-
inverting and vice-versa, according to the sign of the input signal. Figure
A2-5 depicts graphically this principle of operation and Figure A2-6 shows a
schematic diagram of the stage.

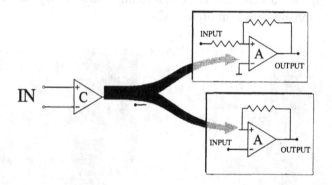

Figure A2-5. Principle of operation of rectifier stage.

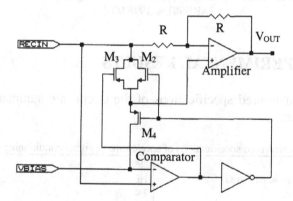

Figure A2-6. Schematic diagram of rectifier stage. From [ARN98], © 1998 IEEE.

This architecture has several features that make it very well suited for
operation at low supply voltage. First it avoids the application of floating p-n
diodes, which are not available in standard Bulk CMOS technologies.
Though they could be replaced by MOS diodes, they have the drawback of
greatly decreasing the signal range that could be handled because even in op-

amp-diode ideal rectifier configurations, the diode forward voltage adds up to the signal at the amplifier's output, which in a 2V power supply context is too high an overhead. Second the switches to be included operate either at the fixed V_{BIAS} voltage (as is the case of M_4 in Figure A2-6) or pass only half of the signal range (M_2 and M_3 in Figure A2-6) thus relaxing the difficulties related to operation at low supply voltage.

Finally, the averaging stage of the block diagram of Figure A2-1, was implemented by an external passive RC low pass filter.

The complete accelerometer conditioning circuit layout and chip microphotograph are shown in Figure A2-7.

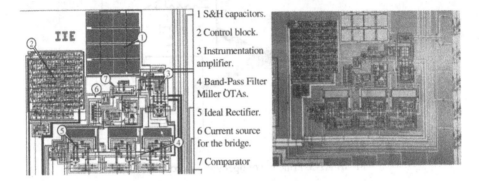

1 S&H capacitors.

2 Control block.

3 Instrumentation amplifier.

4 Band-Pass Filter Miller OTAs.

5 Ideal Rectifier.

6 Current source for the bridge.

7 Comparator

Figure A2-7. Layout and microphotograph of accelerometer signal conditioning circuit. From [ARN98], © 1998 IEEE.

4.   EXPERIMENTAL RESULTS

The main measured specifications of the circuit are summarized in the following table:

Table A2-1. Main measured specifications of accelerometer signal conditioning circuit.

Amplifier Gain	2900
Equivalent input noise (μVrms)	18
Consumption (μA)	3.4
Area (mm^2)	1.82

The total consumption of 3.4μA is divided among the blocks as follows: 0.6μA for the sensor, 0.3μA for the digital control block, 1.45 μA for the band-pass filter amplifier, 0.6 μA for the rectifier stage and 0.45μA in auxiliary stages (bias current branch and voltage buffer for reference voltage).

The minimum measurable acceleration value, corresponding to the measured noise level, resulted to be 0.04g, which is higher than the initial goal but satisfactory for the application purposes.

Finally, Figure A2-8 shows the result of a "field" test of the circuit. In this test, the heart rate of a healthy person doing physical exercise was acquired simultaneously with the output of the circuit. Then, the heart rate that the pacemaker algorithm would set based on the output of the accelerometer circuit was compared with the measured rate of the healthy heart. Figure A2-8 shows the measured output of our circuit (trace C), the measured cardiac frequency of the person (trace A) and the simulated heart rate generated by the pacemaker algorithm fed with the digitized output of our circuit (trace B). The test consisted of different levels of physical activities like walking and running.

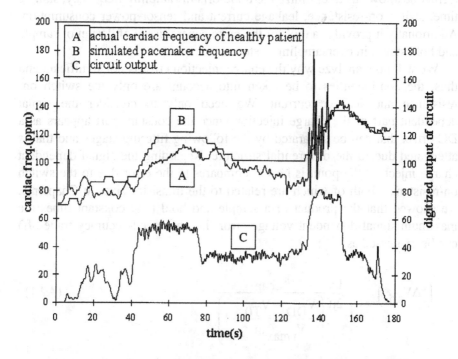

Figure A2-8. Overall "field" performance test of accelerometer conditioning circuit. From [ARN98], © 1998 IEEE.

5.   SAMPLE AND HOLD DESIGN METHODOLOGY

This section describes the results presented in [ARN97].

The power consumption of the sensor interface shown in Figure A2-2 depends on the sampling frequency and sample time (which is related to the time the sensor is on). The signal appearing at the output of the sample and hold is affected by errors due to the switch non-idealities. As we discuss below, the switch non-idealities that are significant in this case are the switch on-resistance and leakage current. These errors are also dependent on the sample time and sampling frequency. In this Section we will present a technique to fully evaluate these effects. We will also show that the traditional approach for estimating the required switch on-resistance (Chapter 8 in [VDP94]), which is based on the objective of a given settling error at the end of the sample time, leads to oversized designs. The proposed technique allows us to optimize the trade-offs in sampling frequency, sample time, switch on-resistance, leakage current and sensor power consumption. Additionally it provides a tool for the more general issue of design of sample and hold stages in oversampling systems.

We will now analyze why the charge injection error is not significant and thus, the non-idealities to be taken into account are only the switch on-resistance and leakage current. We need only to consider the signal dependent part of the charge injection since the constant part appears as a DC offset that can be separated by the following filtering stages and that is attenuated due to the differential structure. Regarding the signal dependent charge injection the point is how it compares to the error due to the switch on-resistance, both of which are related to the transistor size. In Chapter 3, we showed that the product of a sample and hold time constant times the maximum signal dependent voltage error (i.e. the speed-accuracy trade-off) can be expressed as:

$$\left(\tau \Delta V_{s.d.} \right)_{max} = \frac{L^2}{2\mu} \frac{k_{chan}}{\left(\dfrac{V_{DD} - V_{T0}}{V_{i\,max} \cdot n} - 1 \right)} \tag{A2.1}$$

where τ is the switch time constant equal to the product of the on-resistance and the sampling capacitor, $\Delta V_{s.d.}$ is the signal dependent error voltage, L is the channel length, μ is the mobility, k_{chan} is the charge distribution coefficient channel charge to both sides of the switch, V_{DD} the power supply voltage, V_{T0} the threshold voltage, n the body effect coefficient and V_{imax} the maximum signal amplitude to the switch. Therefore this product is independent on the switch width. Since in our application we are dealing with very small signal amplitudes (V_{imax} in the μV range), the resulting $\tau.\Delta V_{s.d.}$ product is very small and the speed-accuracy trade-off is much relaxed. This trade-off is further relaxed by the accurate determination of the requirements on the switch resistance through the method proposed in this section. Hence, the determining factor in this context will be the effect of the switch resistance and not the signal dependent charge injection error as can also be verified a posteriori based on the resulting design.

The switch noise will also be negligible with respect to the amplifiers input noise.

In addition, both noise and charge injection can be accurately estimated with well established models, while, as we show below, in the case of the switch on-resistance and leakage, traditional models lead to highly oversized designs.

The section is organized as follows. First, we present the motivation behind the proposed methodology. We then describe the modeling technique applied for the switch on-resistance. Next, the effect of the leakage currents is added. Finally, we present examples on the current consumption reduction that can be achieved and the validation of the proposed method through simulation and experimental results.

5.1   Motivation

Figure A2-9 shows an intuitive view of the trade-off between sample time (T_{ON}) and sample frequency in relation to the error due to the switch on-resistance. In Figure A2-9 a) we have a low sampling frequency and long sample time so that the sampled signal $x_S(t)$ settles to the input value $x(t)$ with negligible error. In Figure A2-9 b) we suppose higher sampling frequency and a very short sampling time so an important error, due to the incomplete charge of the capacitor, appears when the signal is sampled; however the resulting sampled signal $x_S(t)$ follows the input signal closer than in Figure A2-9 a).

The proposed model of the sample and hold makes it possible to optimize the trade-off depicted in Figure A2-9 by quantifying the influence of the sampling frequency and sample time together with the switch on-resistance and leakage currents.

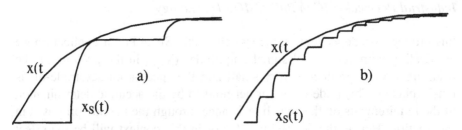

Figure A2-9. Graphic representation of the trade-off between sample time and sampling frequency.

5.2   Sample and hold with switch on-resistance

The proposed model is an extension of the ideal sample & hold model, which is recalled in Figure A2-10 ([OPP83]).

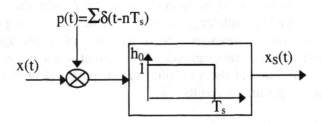

Figure A2-10. Ideal sample and hold model.

This model represents an ideal sample and hold as an ideal sampler, which multiplies the input signal by a Dirac's delta or impulse train, followed by the convolution with the pulse function $h_0(t)$, as expressed in Eq. (A2.2). The effect of the convolution with the pulse function is the holding action of keeping the output at a constant value, equal to the sampled value, during the sampling period T_S.

$$x_S(t) = \sum_{-\infty}^{+\infty} x(t - nT_S).\delta(t - nT_S) * h_0(t) \tag{A2.2}$$

The Fourier transform of $h_0(t)$, noted $H_0(f)$, is given by:

$$h_0(t) \leftrightarrow H_0(f) = T_S . \mathrm{sinc}(\pi f T_S) e^{j\pi f T_S} \tag{A2.3}$$

where sinc() stands for the function $\sin(x)/x$.

Taking Fourier transforms to both sides of Eq. (A2.2), we arrive to the well-known expression of the Fourier transform of the ideal sampled and held signal $X_S(f)$, including the "sinc distortion" factor:

$$X_S(f) = \sin c(\pi f T_S) e^{j\pi f T_S} . \sum_{-\infty}^{+\infty} X(f - nf_S) \tag{A2.4}$$

We will now consider how to include in this model the error associated to the incomplete charge of the sampling capacitor C due to the non-zero on-resistance of the switch.

This can be easily done if we consider the sample time T_{ON} (the time when the switch is on, charging the capacitor C) negligible with respect to the sampling period T_S. This is the case in our accelerometer application since we try to minimize T_{ON} in order to minimize power consumption. In addition, the resulting expression is also a good approximation when this hypothesis does not hold (i.e. T_{ON} is comparable to T_S) and the signal is oversampled. In this case, it can be shown that what we are discarding, when considering T_{ON} to be negligible with respect to T_S, are high frequency components, which are out of the signal band.

Then, under the assumption of T_{ON} negligible, the evolution of the sampled and held signal is as shown in Figure A2-11.

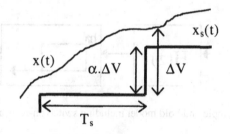

Figure A2-11. Input (x(t)) and sampled and held signal ($x_S(t)$) with on-resistance error when sample time T_{ON} is much smaller than sample period T_S.

The essential issue in order to extend the ideal sample and hold model to include the on-resistance effect is that the sampled and held signal of Figure A2-11 can be determined from the ideally sampled signal through a discrete time filter as shown below.

By taking into account the exponential charge of the capacitor through the R_{ON} switch resistance, $x_S(n.T_S)$ is given by:

$$x_S(nT_S) = x_S((n-1)T_S) + [x(nT_S) - x_S((n-1)T_S)]\left(1 - e^{-T_{ON}/R_{ON}C}\right) \quad \text{(A2.5)}$$

From this expression, ΔV and α shown in Figure A2-11 are given by:

$$\Delta V = x(nT_S) - x_S((n-1)T_S) \text{ and } \alpha = 1 - e^{T_{ON}/R_{ON}C} \quad \text{(A2.6)}$$

Eq. (A2.5) defines a discrete time filter with input $x(n)$ and output $x_s(n)$ that models the effect of the switch on-resistance. Its Z-transform transfer function is given by:

$$H(z) = \frac{X_S(z)}{X(z)} = \frac{\alpha}{1 - z(1-\alpha)} \quad \text{(A2.7)}$$

Then we can proceed in analog way to the ideal sample and hold case, but introducing $H(z)$ as shown in Figure A2-12, to take into account the on-resistance effect.

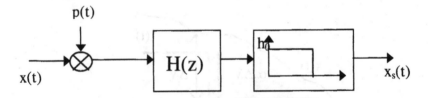

Figure A2-12. Sample and hold model including switch on-resistance effect.

Calculating the frequency response of the digital filter $H(z)$ as $H(e^{jwT_S})$ and applying the model of Figure A2-12, we have the spectrum (Fourier transform) of the output signal $X_S(f)$.

$$X_S(f) = \frac{\alpha}{1 - e^{j2\pi fT_S}(1-\alpha)} \cdot \text{sin } c(\pi fT_S) e^{j\pi fT_S} \cdot \sum_{-\infty}^{+\infty} X(f - nf_S) \quad \text{(A2.8)}$$

The consequences of this improved model can be analyzed considering the relative error in the signal amplitude, noted re and defined as:

$$re(f) = 1 - \frac{|X_S(f)|}{|X(f)|} \tag{A2.9}$$

Figure A2-13 a) plots re as a function of the oversampling ratio defined as f_S/f when the sample/hold duty cycle (T_{ON}/T_S) and the sample and hold time constant $R_{ON}C$ are kept constant. Figure A2-13 a) also shows the relative influence of two factors in re. These are the traditional sinc distortion calculated with Eq. (A2.4) (referred as re_I) and the difference $re_{II} = re - re_I$, which can be seen as the influence in the frequency response of the incomplete settling relative error ε. The voltage relative error ε at the end of the sample period T_{ON} is equal to $(1-\alpha)$ and is plotted in Figure A2-13 b). As the oversampling ratio increases, the error due to the sinc distortion re_I decreases causing re to decrease in spite of the fact that the error ε grows (due to the decrease of T_{ON}), making re_{II} grow. As we can see, about 25% settling error causes only about 5% relative error re in the sampled signal because of the benefits of oversampling. Figure A2-13 a) shows that a good compromise between total error and sampling frequency can be found at f_S/f around 6 to 8 for the particular example. It also shows that taking into account only error ε as error estimate leads to a highly pessimistic estimation.

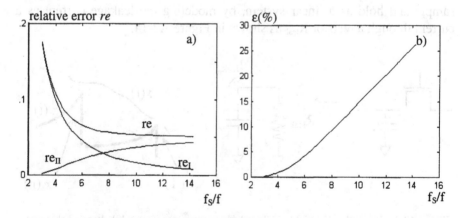

Figure A2-13. Sample and hold error terms as a function of oversampling factor f_S/f for constant sample/hold duty cycle (T_{ON} / T_S). a) total amplitude relative error (re as defined in Eq. (A2.9)), sinc error (re_I) and error difference $re_{II} = re - re_I$. b) voltage settling error $\varepsilon = 1-\alpha$ at the end of sampling time T_{ON}.

Some comments are due on the scope and consequences of this analysis. As discussed in the previous paragraph, two error sources appear when dealing with a sample and hold with switch on-resistance: the sinc factor due to the sample and hold effect and an additional factor related to the incomplete settling during the sample time. In the analysis based on Figure A2-13 what we are doing is to choose the minimum frequency that provides an optimum balance between both error sources and that decreases the total error. It is well known that an appropriate filter, placed after the sample and hold stage, can compensate the sinc factor. However, this compensation implies added consumption and circuit complexity and is not applied in many systems. Furthermore, even when the sinc factor compensation is applied, the resulting error is much less than the ε settling error. This can be understood based on the fact that the settling relative error is taken with respect to the voltage *step* at the output of the sample and hold at each sampling period, which is much smaller than the total output voltage of the sample and hold. The previous discussions are only valid in the case of a sample and hold that, by definition, preserves the previous output value. Similar considerations are not valid when analyzing, for example, the influence of the switch on-resistance in many switched capacitor circuits, where capacitors must be completely charged in one sample period.

5.3   Leakage current effect

The presence of leakage currents makes the capacitor voltage change during the hold phase. This can be taken into account, while preserving the sample and hold as a linear system, by modeling the leakage current as a current through a resistor R_{leak} as shown in Figure A2-14.

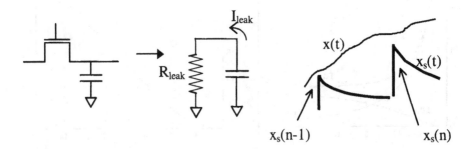

Figure A2-14. Principle of model to include leakage currents effect, while keeping the model to be linear.

This approach neglects the non-linear dependence of leakage currents with the sample and hold output voltage. In the case of our accelerometer circuit this effect is in fact negligible since we have a very small AC signal plus a DC bias value. Hence the leakage currents will be determined by the almost fixed total (DC plus AC) value and will be approximately constant. In this case the R_{leak} value can be suitably chosen as equal to V/I_{leak}, where V is the voltage DC bias value and I_{leak} is the leakage current which correspond to this bias voltage. In a more general case this approach seems to be a good first order approximation to the problem.

Applying the principle shown in Figure A2-14, the effect of leakage currents can be included in the model of Figure A2-12. This is done by modifying the digital filter $H_2(z)$ to include the effect of the changing voltage during the hold phase and replacing the rectangular pulse $h_0(t)$ by an exponential pulse $h_1(t)$ equal to $e^{-t/Rleak.C}$ for t between 0 and T_S. This exponential pulse is the result of the evolution of the output voltage during the hold phase.

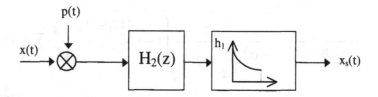

Figure A2-15. Model that includes the leakage currents effect.

We will now deduce the expressions of the filter H_2 and the resulting spectrum of the sampled and held signal. For $nT_S < t < (n+1)T_S$, the effect of the leakage resistor leads to:

$$x_s(t) = x_s(nT_s)e^{-\left(t - nT_s\right)/R_{leak}C} \qquad (A2.10)$$

Proceeding as in the case of the model for the on-resistance, we include both effects on the discrete signal $x_s[n]$ in a discrete time filter:

$$x_S[n] = \alpha(x[n] - \beta x_S[n-1]) - \beta x_S[n-1]$$
$$\text{with } \beta = e^{-T_s/R_{leak}C} \qquad (A2.11)$$

Applying the Z transform, the following expression results for $H_2(z)$:

$$H_2(z) = \frac{\alpha}{1 - \beta(1-\alpha)z} \qquad (A2.12)$$

To obtain the expression of the continuous time $x_S(t)$ signal we make a convolution with an exponential pulse $h_1(t)$. This convolution affects the spectrum of $x_S(t)$ with the following factor:

$$h_1(t) = e^{-t/\tau}, \tau = R_{leak}C \Rightarrow$$

$$h_1(f) = \frac{1}{\frac{1}{\tau} + j2\pi f}\left(1 - e^{-\left[\frac{1}{\tau} + j2\pi f\right]T_S}\right)$$

(A2.13)

The resulting expression for the spectrum of $x_S(t)$, taking into account both , the on-resistance and leakage current effects is:

$$X_S(f) = \frac{\alpha}{1 - \beta.e^{j2\pi f T_S}(1 - \alpha)} \cdot \frac{1}{\left(\frac{1}{\tau} + j2\pi f\right)}\left(1 - e^{-\left(\frac{1}{\tau} + j2\pi f\right)T_S}\right)\frac{1}{T_S}\sum_{-\infty}^{+\infty}X(f - nf_S)$$

(A2.14)

5.4   A synthesis example

We will take an example from our piezoresistive accelerometer interface circuit. There we use a pMOS transistor to sample a small signal of $500\mu V$ amplitude around a common mode voltage of 1.75V with 2V power supply. The frequency of interest ranges from 0.5Hz to 7Hz. Sampling frequency f_S was fixed at 125Hz and capacitor C is 35 pF. We want to minimize power consumption, and to do so we must minimize T_{ON}, which is related to the time that the sensor is on. We want our signal amplitude to have an error of less than 1% in the band of interest. The estimated on-resistance of the switch for the 1.75V input voltage is $50k\Omega$ (worst case value) and leakage currents are 22fA considering 25% mismatch, as suggested in [SHO86], between leakage currents of the differential sample and hold.

With these data and applying Eq. (A2.14), we obtain the attenuation in the input signal due to the sample and hold. Figure A2-16 shows the attenuation at the maximum signal frequency of 7Hz as a function of the sample time T_{ON}. From this plot we see that T_{ON} equal to $4.7\mu s$ fulfills the 1% error requirement.

If we apply a rough criterion of assuring a settling error ε of 1% for the $R_{ON}C$ circuit we would have T_{ON} equal $8.1\mu s$ that doubles the actually required time and therefore consumption.

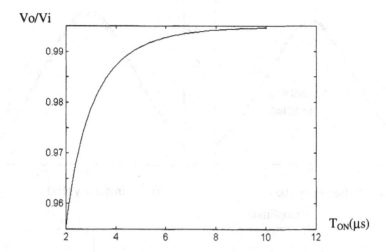

Figure A2-16. Amplitude transfer function for a sampled 7Hz signal as a function of T_{ON}.

5.5   Simulation and experimental results

Simulation and experimental measurements were done to check the proposed model. The sample and hold tested was implemented with a Bulk nMOS transistor with W equal to 40µm and L equal to 12µm. Sampling frequency f_S is 125Hz and power supply 3V. The capacitor C and T_{ON} values were taken so as to make the studied effects clearly visible. A 100nF capacitor and 400µs T_{ON} were applied. Following the sample and hold was placed a low pass filter to cut frequency components above the sampling frequency.

Simulations

Simulations were made using the EKV model ([VIT93, ENZ95]) for the nMOS transistor. The input signal was a sine wave of variable frequency, 400mV AC amplitude and 200mV DC value. Three simulations are shown in Figure A2-17. In the first one, leakage currents are not simulated, while in second one they are simulated placing a 500kΩ resistor in parallel with the sample and hold capacitor. In both plots theoretical and simulated curves are shown with high agreement. The third plot shows the predicted and simulated transfer functions when leakage currents are modeled in the simulator through a reverse biased diode connected in parallel with the sampling capacitor. For this case our predictions resulted in a small overestimation of the leakage current and on-resistance effects in the sample and hold performance. This difference is due to the assumption of a linear behavior of the leakage current effect.

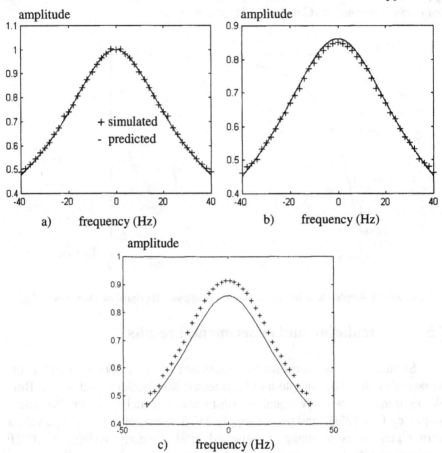

Figure A2-17. Simulated (+ symbols) and predicted (solid line) transfer functions for a sample and hold with no leakage current (a)), leakage currents simulated with a resistor (b)) and leakage currents simulated with a reverse connected diode (c)).

Measurements

The measured value of R_{ON} was 3.4kΩ. The corresponding settling error ε, previously defined, is 0.32. Figure A2-18 plots the predicted transfer function, the measured transfer function and the sinc transfer function given by Eq. A2.4. Leakage effects were expected to be negligible and were not measurable.

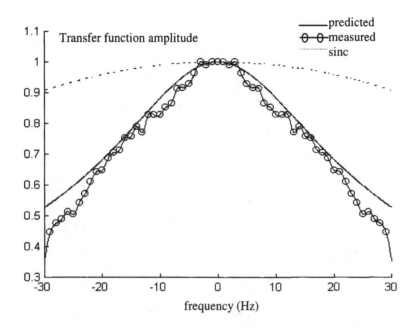

Figure A2-18. Predicted (solid line) and measured (circles) transfer function of a sample and hold, shown together with the sinc function (dashed line).

The simulation and experimental results show very good agreement with the proposed model.

6. CONCLUSIONS

We have proposed a new modeling technique for a sample and hold stage, particularly in an oversampling environment. This technique makes it possible to precisely take into account the effect of the switch on-resistance and leakage currents on the stage operation. We have provided a model, the resulting expressions for the spectrum of the non-ideal sampled and held signal, and have connected these mathematical results with intuitive visualizations of what happens in the time domain. The application of these tools makes it possible to either relax the requirements on the switch on-resistance or, in our application, to optimize the sensor interface to minimize power consumption.

Bibliography

[ADA79] R. Adams, "Filtering in the log domain", Preprint 1470, *63rd Audio Engineering Society Conference*, New York, May 1979.

[ADA95] J. Adam, "Wilson Greatbatch", *IEEE Spectrum*, March 1995, pp. 56- 61.

[AKI98] T. Akin, K. Najafi, "A Wireless Implantable Multichannel Digital Neural Recording System for a Micromachined Sieve Electrode", *IEEE Journal of Solid-State Circuits*, vol 33, no. 1, Jan. 1998, pp. 109-118.

[ALL84] P.E. Allen, E. Sánchez-Sinencio, *Switched Capacitor Circuits*, New York, Van Nostrand Reinhold, 1984, pp. 429 - 437.

[ARN97] A. Arnaud, F. Silveira, "The design methodology of a sample and hold for a low-power sensor interface circuit", *Proceedigns of the X Brazilian Symposium on Integrated Circuit Design*, Gramado, Brasil, August 1997, pp. pp. 243 - 252.

[ARN98] A. Arnaud, M. Barú, G. Picún, F. Silveira, "Design of a Micropower Signal Conditioning Circuit for a Piezoresistive Acceleration Sensor", *Proceedings of the 1998 IEEE ISCAS (International Symposium in Circuits and Systems)*, Monterey, USA, Vol. I, pp. 269 - 272.

[BAR96] M. Barú, O. de Oliveira, F. Silveira, "A 2V Rail-to-Rail Micropower CMOS Comparator", *Journal of Solid-State Devices and Circuits, Brazilian Microelectronics Society*, Feb. 1997, Vol. 5, No. 1, pp. 9 – 13 and *Proceedings of the XI Conference of the Brazilian Microelectronics Society*, Aguas de Lindoia, Brasil, July 29 - August 2, 1996, pp. 121 - 126.

[BAR98] M. Barú, H. Valdenegro, C. Rossi, F. Silveira, "An ASK Demodulator in CMOS Technology", *Proceedings of the IV Iberchip Workshop*, Mar del Plata, Argentina, 1998, pp. 37-42.

[BAS01] A. Baschirotto, D. Bijno; R. Castello; F. Montecchi, "A 1V 1.2μW 4th order bandpass switched-opamp SC filter for a cardiac pacer sensing stage", *Proceedings of the 2001 IEEE ISCAS (International Symposium in Circuits and Systems)*, Geneva, Switzerland, Vol. 3, pp. 173 - 176.

[BRA98] R. Braham, "Medical Electronics. Implanted pulse generator quells tremor", *IEEE Spectrum*, January 1998, pp. 62-66.

[CAR75] A. B. Carlson, *Communication Systems*, 2nd Ed. New York, McGraw-Hill, 1975.

[CAS851]   R. Castello and P. Gray, "Performance Limitations in Switched-Capacitor
           Filters", *IEEE Transactions on Circuits and Systems*, vol. 32, Sep. 1985, pp.865-
           876.
[CAS852]   R. Castello, P. Gray, "A High-Performance Micropower Switched-Capacitor
           Filter", *IEEE Journal of Solid-State Circuits*, vol SC-20, Dec. 1985, pp. 1122-
           1132.
[CAS92]   R. Castello, "CMOS Buffer Amplifiers" in *Analog Circuit Design:*
           Operational Amplifiers, Analog to Digital Converters, Analog Computer Aided
           Design, edited by J. Huijsing. R. van de Plassche and W. Sansen, Kluwer
           Academic Publishers, Dordrecht, 1992
[CCC03]   Centro de Construcción de Cardioestimuladores del Uruguay S.A.,
           http://www.ccc.com.uy.
[CCC96]   Centro de Construcción de Cardioestimuladores del Uruguay S.A., Specifications
           of integrated circuit for pacemaker, *Technical annex of Contract with*
           Universidad de la República, Montevideo, Uruguay, 1996.
[CEN00]   CEN/CENELEC, *Standard prEN 45502: Active Implantable Medical Devices*,
           September 2000.
[CHU82]   C. T. Chuang, "Analysis of the settling behavior of an operational amplifier,"
           IEEE Journal of Solid-State Circuits, vol. SC-17, pp. 74-80, Feb. 1982.
[COL91]   J. P. Colinge, *Silicon-on-Insulator Technology: Materials to VLSI*, Kluwer
           Academic Publishers, 1991.
[CRO94]   J. Crols, M. Steyaert, "Switched-Opamp: An Approach to Realize Full CMOS
           Switched-Capacitor Circuits at Very Low Power Supply Voltages", *IEEE Journal*
           of Solid-State Circuits, vol. 29, No. 8, Aug. 94, pp.936..942.
[CUN98]   A. Cunha, M. Schneider, C. Galup-Montoro, "An MOS transistor model for
           analog circuit design", *IEEE Journal of Solid-State Circuits*, vol. 33, pp. 1510-
           1519, Oct. 1998.
[CUP79]   R. Cuppens, H. De Man, W. Sansen, "Simulation of Large On-Chip Capacitors
           and Inductors", *IEEE Journal of Solid-State Circuits*, vol. 14, pp. 543 - 547, June
           1979.
[DEG82]   M. Degrauwe, J. Rijmenants, E. Vittoz, H. DeMan, "Adaptive Biasing CMOS
           Amplifiers", *IEEE Journal of Solid-State Circuits*, vol SC-17, Jun. 1982, pp.
           522-528.
[EGG98]   J. P. Eggermont, *Study and Realization of SOI Operational Amplifiers for High-*
           Temperature or High-Frequency Applications, PhD. Thesis, Université
           Catholique de Louvain, Louvain-la-Neuve, Belgium, 1998.
[ENZ95]   C.C. Enz, F.K. Krummenacher and E.A. Vittoz, "An Analytical MOS Transistor
           Model Valid in All Regions of Operation and Dedicated to Low-Voltage and
           Low-Current Applications", *Analog Integrated Circuits and Signal Processing*,
           No. 8, pp. 83 - 114, 1995, Kluwer Academic Publishers.
[ENZ98]   C. Enz, M. Punzenberger, "1-V Log-Domain Filters", in *Analog Circuit Design*,
           Ed. by W. Sansen, R. Van de Plassche and J. Huijsing, 1998, Kluwer Academic
           Publishers.
[ESC95]   R. Eschauzier, J. Huijsing, *Frequency compensation techniques for low-power*
           operational amplifiers, Kluwer Academic Publishers, Dordrecht, 1995.
[EUR01]   Europractice, *2001 Annual Report*, available online at:
           http://www.europractice.imec.be/europractice/on-line-docs/homepage/Annual_
           report_2001.pdf

[FER97]   G. Ferri, W. Sansen et al, "A Rail-to-Rail Constant-gm Low-Voltage CMOS
          Operational Transconductance Amplifier", *IEEE Journal of Solid-State Circuits*,
          vol. 32, Oct. 1997, pp. 1563-1567.

[FIA88]   O. Fiandra, "The First Pacemaker Implant in America", *PACE*, Vol. 11, August
          1988, pp. 1234 – 1238, Futura Publishing Company.

[FLA01]   D. Flandre et al, "Fully-depleted SOI CMOS technology for heterogeneous
          micropower, high-temperature or RF microsystems", *Solid-State Electronics*, 45
          (2001) 541-549.

[FLA94]   D. Flandre, J.P Eggermont, D. De Ceuster, P. Jespers, "Comparison of SOI versus
          bulk performances of CMOS micropower single-stage OTAs", *Electronics
          Letters* 30, pp. 1933-1934, 1994.

[FLA96]   D. Flandre, L. Ferreira, P. Jespers and J. P. Colinge, "Modeling and application of
          fully-depleted SOI MOSFETs for low-voltage low-power analog CMOS
          circuits", *Solid-State Electronics*, 39, pp. 455 – 460, 1996.

[FLA99]   Flandre D., Colinge J.P., Chen J., De Ceuster D., Eggermont J.P., Ferreira L.,
          Gentinne B., Jespers P.G.A., Viviani A., Gillon R., Raskin J.P., Vander Vorst A.,
          Vanhoenacker D., Silveira F., "Fully-Depleted SOI CMOS Technology for Low-
          Voltage Low-Power Mixed Digital/Analog/Microwave Circuits", *Analog
          Integrated Circuits and Signal Processing*, Special Section on Low Voltage/Low
          Power Design, Vol. 21, No. 3 Dec. 1999, pp. 213 – 228, Kluwer Academic Press.

[FOR94]   F. Forti and M.E. Wright, "Measurement of MOS Current Mismatch in the Weak
          Inversion Region", *IEEE Journal of Solid-State Circuits* , Vol. 29, pp. 138-142,
          Feb. 1994.

[FRE93]   D. Frey, "Log Domain Filtering: An Approach to Current Mode Filtering", *IEE
          Proc. G*, vol. 140, pp. 406-416, Dec. 1993.

[GAO92]   M. Gao, J.P. Colinge, L. Lauwers, S. Wu and C. Claeys, "Twin-MOSFET
          Structure for Suppression of Kink and Parasitic Bipolar Effects in SOI MOSFETs
          at Room and Liquid Helium Temperatures", *Solid-State Electronics*, Vol. 35, No.
          4, 1992, pp. 505-512.

[GAR77]   P. Garde, "Transconductance Cancellation for Operational Amplifiers", *IEEE
          Journal of Solid-State Circuits*, vol. 12, pp. 310 - 311, June 1977.

[GED90]   L. Geddes, "Historical Highlights in Cardiac Pacing", *IEEE Engineering in
          Medicine and Biology*, June 1990, pp. 12-18.

[GER00]   A. Gerosa, A. Novo, A. Neviani, "A low-power sensing and digitization of
          cardiac signals based on sigma-delta conversion", *Proceedings of ISLPED '00
          (International Symposium on Low Power Electronics and Design, 2000)*, Rapallo,
          Italy, pp. 216-218.

[GER011] A. Gerosa, A. Novo, A. Mengalli, A. Neviani, "A micro-power low noise log-
          domain amplifier for the sensing chain of a cardiac pacemaker", *Proceedings of
          the 2001 IEEE ISCAS (International Symposium in Circuits and Systems)*,
          Sydney, Australia, Vol. I, pp. 296 - 299.

[GER012] A. Gerosa; A. Novo and A. Neviani, "An analog front-end for the acquisition of
          biomedical signals, fully integrated in a 0.8 μm CMOS process", *Proceedings of
          the 2001 Southwest Symposium on Mixed-Signal Design (SSMSD)*, 25-27 Feb.
          2001, Austin, TX, USA, pp. 152 – 157.

[GRA93]   P. Gray, R. Meyer, *Analysis and Design of Analog Integrated Circuits*, 3rd
          Edition, John Wiley and Sons, 1993.

[GRE03]   Wilson Greatbatch Ltd., http://www.greatbatch.com. Last visited 9th. July, 2003.

[GRE86]   R. Gregorian, G.C. Temes, *Analog MOS Integrated Circuits for Signal Processing*, New York, John Wiley & Sons, 1986.

[GRI97]   R. Griffith, R. Vyne, R. Dotson, T. Petty, "A 1-V BiCMOS Rail-to-Rail Amplifier with n-Channel Depletion Mode Input Stage", *IEEE Journal of Solid-State Circuits*, Vol. 32, No. 12, Dec. 1997, pp. 2012 - 2023.

[GUI03]   Guidant Corporation, "Pulsar Max II pacemaker product information", available online at: http://www.guidant.com/products/pulsar2.shtml. Last visited 4th May, 2003.

[HEL99]   A. Heller, "Implanted Electrochemical Glucose Sensors for the Management of Diabetes" in *Annual Review of Biomedical Engineering*, 1999, Annual Reviews.

[HOS85]   B. Hosticka, "Performance comparisons of analog and digital circuits", *Proceedings of the IEEE*, vol. 73, pp. 25-29, Jan. 1985.

[HUI85]   J.H. Huijsing, D. Linebarger, "Low-voltage operational amplifier with rail-to-rail input and output ranges", *IEEE Journal of Solid-State Circuits*, vol. SC-20, pp. 1144-1150, Dec. 1985.

[IBM011]   IBM Corp., "Silicon-on-insulator (SOI)", avalaible online at http://www-3.ibm.com/chips/bluelogic/showcase/soi/. Last visited, 9th July, 2003.

[IBM012]   IBM Corp., "IBM introduces 1 GHz PowerPC microprocessor, First chips to use copper, SOI and low-k, East Fishkill, NY - October 17, 2001", available online at http://www-3.ibm.com/chips/news/2001/1017_750fx.html, Last visited, 9th July, 2003.

[ICS00]   ICSensors, *Accel. 3022 and 3028:OEM Accelerometer Piezoresistive Low Cost, Data Sheet*, April 2000.

[ITR01]   International Technology Roadmap for Semiconductors, 2001 Edition, Section on Process Integration, Devices, Structures and Emerging Research Devices, p. 31, Non classical CMOS, available online at: http://public.itrs.net/Files/2001ITRS/Home.htm, Last visited, 9th July, 2003.

[JOH97]   D. Johns, K. Martin, *Analog Integrated Circuit Design*, John Wiley and Sons, New York, 1997.

[KAM74]   B. Y. Kamath, R. G. Meyer, and P. R. Gray, "Relationship between frequency response and settling time of operational amplifiers", *IEEE Journal of Solid-State Circuits*, vol. SC-9, pp. 347-352, Dec.1974.

[KRI01]   N. Krishnapura, Y. Tsividis, "Noise and Power Reduction in Filters Through the Use of Adjustable Biasing", *IEEE Journal of Solid-State Circuits*, Vol. 36, No. 12, Dec 2001, pp. 1912 - 1920.

[KRU81]   F. Krummenacher, "High Voltage Gain CMOS OTA for Micropower SC Filters", *Electronics Letters*, Vol. 17, No. 4, pp. 160-162, 19th Feb. 1981.

[LAK94]   K. Laker, W. Sansen, *Design of Analog Integrated Circuits and Systems*, Mc Graw Hill, New York, 1994.

[LAM92]   M. Lambrechts, W. Sansen, *Biosensors: Microelectrochemical Devices*, Institute of Physics Publishing, Bristol, 1992.

[LAN97]   K. de Langen, J Huijsing, "Compact 1.8V Low-Power CMOS Operational Amplifier Cells for VLSI", *Proc. IEEE ISSCC 1997*, pp. 346-347.

[LAN99]   K. de Langen, J. Huijsing, *Compact Low-Voltage and High-Speed CMOS, BiCMOS and Bipolar Operational Amplifiers*, Kluwer Academic Publishers, Dordrecht, 1999.

[LEN01]   L. Lentola, A. Mozzi, A. Neviani, A. Baschirotto, "A 1μA Front-End for Pacemaker Atrial Sensing Channels", *Proceedings ESSCIRC 01*, Austria, Sep. 2001.

[LIN86]   I. C. Lin and J. H. Nevin, "A modified time-domain model for nonlinear analysis of an operational amplifier," *IEEE Journal of Solid-State Circuits*, vol. SC-21,. pp. 478-483, June 1986.

[MAR81]   K. Martin, A. Sedra, "Effects of the Op Amp Finite Gain and Bandwidth on the Performance of Switched-Capacitor Filters", *IEEE Trans. on Circuits and Systems*, vol. 28, pp. 822 – 829, Aug. 1981.

[MAR87]   K. Martin, L. Ozcolak, Y. Lee, G. Temes, "A Differential Switched-Capacitor Amplifier", *IEEE Journal of Solid-State Circuits*, Vol. SC 22, no. 1, pp.104- 106, Feb. 1987

[MAT87]   H. Matsumoto, K. Watanabe, "Spike-Free Switched-Capacitor Circuits", *Electronics Letters*, Vol. 23, no.8, pp. 428-429, April 1987.

[MCC75]   J. L. McCreary and P. R. Gray, "All MOS charge redistribution analog-to-digital conversion techniques -- Part I", *IEEE Journal of Solid-State Circuits*, vol SC-10, pp. 371 - 379, Dec. 1975.

[MOO01]   S. Moore, "New Breed of Pacemaker Addresses Heart Failure", *IEEE Spectrum*, Oct. 2001, pp. 30-33.

[NAG89]   K. Nagaraj, "A Parasitic-Insensitive Area-Efficient Approach to Realizing Very Large Time Constants in Switched-Capacitor Circuits", *IEEE Transactions on Circuits and Systems*, Vol. 36, No.9, pp. 1210 – 1216, Sep. 1989.

[NG99]   H. Ng, R. Ziazadeh, D. J. Allstot, "A Multistage Amplifier Technique with Embedded Frequency Compensation", *IEEE Journal of Solid-State Circuits*, Vol. 34, No. 3, March 1999, pp. 339 – 347.

[NOV01]   A. Novo, A. Gerosa, A. Neviani, "A Sub-Micron CMOS Programmable Charge Pump for Implantable Pacemaker", *Analog Integrated Circuits and Signal Processing*, Vol. 27, 2001, pp. 211 – 217, Kluwer Academic Press.

[NOV99]   A. Novo, A. Gerosa, A. Neviani, A. Mozzi, E. Zanoni. "Programmable voltage multiplier for pacemaker output pulse generation", *Electronics Letters*, Volume: 35 Issue: 7, pp. 560 – 561, 1 April 1999

[OPP83]   A. Oppenheim, A. Willsky, I. Young, *Signals and Systems*, Prentice Hall, New Jersey, 1983.

[PAR98]   J. Parramon, F. Silveira, P. Doguet, D. Marin, M. Verleysen, J. Arzuaga, E. Valderrama, "Implantable Telemetry Microsystem for Recording Purposes", *IV Workshop de Iberchip*, Mar del Plata, Argentina, Marzo de 1998, pgs. 351 - 357.

[PEL89]   M. Pelgrom, A. Duinmaijer, A. Welbers, "Matching Properties of MOS Transistors", *IEEE Journal of Solid-State Circuits*, Vol. 24, No. 5, Oct. 1989, pp. 1433-1440.

[POR98]   L. Portmann, C. Lallement, F. Krummenhacher, "A high density integrated test matrix of MOS transistors for matching study", *Proc. ICMTS*, Kanazawa, Japan, March, 1998.

[RAY98]   C.Raynaud et al., "Fully-depleted 0.25um SOI devices for low power RF mixed analog-digital circuits", *Proc. IEEE International SOI Conference*, Stuart, FL., pp. 67-68, Oct. 1998.

[REY97]   S. Reynolds, "A DC-DC Converter for Short-Channel CMOS Technologies", *IEEE Journal of Solid-State Circuits*, vol. 32, No. 1, January 1997, pp. 111- 113.

[RIT98]   P. Ritter, S. Cazeau, A. Lazarus, "Advanced Programming and New Automatic Functions of Dual-Chamber Pacemakers" in *Recent Advances in Cardiac Pacing Goals for the 21st Century*, Ed. by S. Serge Barold and Jacques Mugida, Futura Publishing Company, Armonk, N.Y., 1998.

[RUS72]   R.W. Russell, T. Frederiksen, "Automotive and Industrial Building Blocks", *IEEE Journal of Solid-State Circuits*, vol. 7, pp. 446-454, Dec. 1972.

[SAC87]   E. Sackinger, W. Guggenbuhl, "A Versatile Building Block: The CMOS Differential Difference Amplifier", *IEEE Journal of Solid-State Circuits*, vol. 22, no. 2, April 1987, pp. 287-294.

[SAN84]   W. Sansen and P. Van Peteghem, "An Area-Efficient Approach to the Design of Very-Large Time Constants in Switched-Capacitor Integrators", *IEEE Journal of Solid-State Circuits*, vol. 19, pp. 772 - 780, October 1984.

[SAN96]   R. Sanders, M. Lee, "Implantable Pacemakers", *Proceedings of the IEEE*, Vol. 84, No. 3, March 1996, pp. 480 – 486.

[SAR97]   R. Sarpeshkar, R. Lyon and C. Mead, "A Low-Power Wide-Linear-Range Transconductance Amplifier", *Analog Integrated Circuits and Signal Processing*, Vol. 13, pp. 123 – 151, 1997, Kluwer Academic Press.

[SED78]   A. Sedra, P. Bracket, *Filter Theory and Design: Active and Passive*, Matrix Publishers Inc. Beaverton, USA, 1978.

[SEE90]   E. Seevinck, "Companding current mode integrator: A new circuit principle for continuous-time monolithic filters", *Electronics Letters*, vol. 26, pp. 2046-2047, Nov. 1990.

[SHO86]   F. Shoucair, " Design Considerations in High Temperature Analog CMOS Integrated Circuits", *IEEE Transactions on Components, Hybrids and Manufacturing Technology*, Vol. CHMT-9, No. 3, Sep. 1986. pp. 242 - 251.

[SHU94]   M. Shultz, R. Rhodes, S. Updike, B. Gilligan, W. Reining, "A Telemetry-Instrumentation System for Monitoring Multiple Subcutaneously Implanted Glucose Sensors", *IEEE Trans. on Biomedical Engineering*, vol. 41, No. 10, pp. 937-942, Oct. 1994.

[SIL00]   F. Silveira, D. Flandre, "Analysis and Design of a Family of Low-Power Class AB Operational Amplifiers", *Proceeedings of the XIII Simposium on Integrated Circuits and Systems Design*, IEEE Computer Press, Manaus, Brasil, September 2000, pp. 94-98.

[SIL021] F. Silveira, D. Flandre, "A 110 nA Pacemaker Sensing Channel in CMOS on Silicon-on-Insulator", *Proceedings of the 2002 IEEE International Symposium on Circuits and Systems (ISCAS 2002)*, 26 to 29 May 2002, Scottsdale, USA, Vol. 5, pp. 181-184.

[SIL022] F. Silveira, D. Flandre, "Operational Amplifier Power Optimization for a Given Total (Slewing plus Linear) Settling Time", *Proceeedings of the XV Simposium on Integrated Circuits and Systems Design*, IEEE Computer Press, Porto Alegre, Brasil, September 2002, pp. 247-253.

[SIL96]   F. Silveira, D. Flandre, P. Jespers, "A gm/ID Based Methodology for the Design of CMOS Analog Circuits and its Application to the Synthesis of a Silicon-on-Insulator Micropower OTA", *IEEE Journal of Solid State Circuits*, Vol. 31, No. 9, Sept. 1996, pp. 1314 - 1319.

[SIL97]   J. Silva-Martínez and J. Salcedo-Suñer, "IC Voltage to Current Transducers with Very Small Transconductance", *Analog Integrated Circuits and Signal Processing*, Vol. 13, pp. 285 – 293, 1997.

[SJO99]   H. Sjoland, *Highly Linear Integrated Wideband Amplifiers*, Kluwer Academic Publishers, Dordrecht, 1999.

[STE87]   M. Steyaert, W. Sansen, C. Zhongyuan, "A micropower low-noise monolithic instrumentation amplifier for medical purposes", *IEEE Journal of Solid-State Circuits*, vol. SC-22, no. 6, pp. 1163-1168, Dec. 1987.

[STO891]   L. Stotts, "Introduction to Implantable Biomedical IC Design", *IEEE Circuits and Devices Magazine*, pp. 12-18, January 1989.

[STO892]   L. J. Stotts, K. R. Infinger, J. Babka, and D. Genzer, "An 8-bit microcomputer with analog subsystems for implantable biomedical application", *IEEE Journal of Solid-State Circuits*, vol. 24, pp. 292 - 300, April 1989.

[TAY94]   R. Taylor, "Switched Capacitor Filters" in *Analog Circuit Design: Low-Power Low-Voltage, Integrated Filters and Smart Power*, Kluwer Academic Publishers, Dordrecht, 1994.

[TEM80]   G. Temes, "Finite Amplifier Gain and Bandwidth Effects in Switched-Capacitor Filters", *IEEE Journal of Solid-State Circuits*, vol. 15, pp. 358-361, June 1980.

[TEM96]   G. Temes, "Simple Formula for Estimation of Minimum Clock-Feedthrough Error Voltage", *Electronics Letters*, 25th Sep. 1986, vol 22, pp. 1069-1070.

[TUR83]   C. Turchetti, G. Masetti, "A Macromodel for Integrated All-MOS Operational Amplifiers", *IEEE Journal of Solid-State Circuits*, vol. SC-18,. pp. 389-394, Aug. 1983.

[VDP94]   R. van de Plassche, *Integrated Analog-to-Digital and Digital-to-Analog Converters*, Kluwer Academic Publishers, Boston, 1994.

[VER96]   M. Verbeck, C. Zimmermann, H. Fiedler, "A MOS Switched-Capacitor Ladder Filter in SIMOX Technology for High Temperature Applications up to 300°C", *IEEE Journal of Solid-State Circuits*, Vol. 31, No. 7, July 1996, pp. 908 -914.

[VIT02]   E. Vittoz and Y. Tsividis, "Frequency-Dynamic Range-Power", in *Trade-Offs in Analog Circuit Design*, ed. by C. Toumazou, G. Moschytz and B. Gilbert, Kluwer Academic Publishers, 2002.

[VIT77]   E. Vittoz, J. Fellrath, "CMOS analog integrated circuits based on weak inversion operation", *IEEE Journal of Solid-State Circuits*, Vol SC-12, pp. 224-231, June 1997.

[VIT90]   E. Vittoz, "Future of analog in the VLSI environment", *Proc. IEEE ISCAS'90*, pp. 1372-1375, New Orleans, 1990.

[VIT93]   E.A. Vittoz, "Micropower Techniques " in *Design of VLSI Circuits for Telecommunications and Signal Processing*, Eds. J.E. Franca and Y.P. Tsividis, Prentice Hall, 1993.

[VIT95]   E. Vittoz, "Low-power low-voltage limitations and prospects in analog design", in *Analog Circuit Design*, Eds. R. Van de Plassche, W. Sansen and J. Huijsing, pp. 3-15, Kluwer 1995.

[VON82]   D. Von Grunigen, R. Sigg, M. Ludwig, U. Brugger, G. Moschytz and H. Melchior, "Integrated switched-capacitor low-pass filter with combined anti-aliasing decimation filter for low frequencies", *IEEE Journal of Solid-State Circuits*, vol. 17, pp. 1024-1028, Dec. 1982.

[WAN95]   F. Wang, R. Harjani, An Improved Model for the Slewing Behavior of Opamps, *IEEE Trans. on Circuits and Systems II*, vol. 42. pp. 679 – 681, Oct. 1995.

[WAR96]   J. Warren, R. Dreher, R. Haworsky, J. Putzke, R. Russie, "Implantable Cardioverter Defibrillators", *Proceedings of the IEEE*, Vol. 84, No. 3, March 1996, pp. 468 – 479.

[WEB951]   J. Webster, *Design of Cardiac Pacemakers*, IEEE Press, Piscataway, NJ ,1995.

[WEB952]   J. Webster, *Medical Instrumentation. Application and Design*, Sec. 1.4 , Medical Measurements Constraints, John Wiley and Sons, New York, 1995.

[WEG87]   G. Wegman, E. Vittoz, F. Rahali, "Charge injection in Analog MOS Switches", *IEEE Journal of Solid-State Circuits*, vol 22, No. 6, Dec. 87, pp. 1091-1097.

[WEI70]   G. Weil, W. L. Engl, and A. Renz, "Integrated pacemakers", *IEEE Journal of Solid-State Circuits*, vol. 5, pp. 67 - 73, April 1970.

[WIL91]   J. Williams, *Analog Design: Art, Science and Personalities*, Butterworth-Heinemann, 1991

[YOU97]   F. You, S. Embabi, and E. Sanchez-Sinencio, "Multistage Amplifier Topologies with Nested Gm-C Compensation", *IEEE Journal of Solid-State Circuits*, vol. 32, Dec. 1997, pp. 2000-2011.

Index